YOU
and
YOUR
BUMP

YOU
and
YOUR
BUMP

Simple steps to pregnancy well-being

Emma Cannon

with Kate Adams

RODALE

This edition first published 2011 by Rodale
an imprint of Pan Macmillan, a division of Macmillan Publishers Ltd
Pan Macmillan, 20 New Wharf Road, London N1 9RR
Basingstoke and Oxford
Associated companies throughout the world
www.panmacmillan.com

ISBN 978-1-9057-4488-6

3 5 7 9 8 6 4

A CIP catalogue record for this book is available from the British Library.

Book designed and set by seagulls.net
Illustrations by Juliet Percival
www.julietpercival.co.uk

Printed and bound by CPI Group (UK) Ltd, Croydon, CR0 4YY

This book is intended as a reference volume only, not as a medical manual.
The information given here is designed to help you make informed decisions
about your health. It is not intended as a substitute for any treatment that you
may have been prescribed by your doctor. If you suspect you have a
medical problem, we urge you to seek competent medical help.

Mention of specific companies, organizations or authorities in this book does not
imply endorsement of the publisher, nor does mention of specific companies,
organizations or authorities in the book imply that they endorse the book.

Addresses, websites and telephone numbers given in this book
were correct at the time of going to press.

Visit **www.panmacmillan.com** to read more about all our books and to buy them.
You will also find features, author interviews and news of any author events, and you can
sign up for e-newsletters so that you're always first to hear about our new releases.

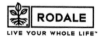

We inspire and enable people to improve their lives and the world around them

For Ali Marling, because she understood
that the meaning of life is love.

Mothers hold their children's hands for a while . . .
their hearts they hold for ever.

contents

foreword
BY DR DONALD GIBB

While the biology of pregnancy and birth has always fascinated me, it is clear that modern medicine cannot provide answers to all the questions, and that treating someone is not always as straightforward as simply addressing and managing diseases. This understanding has increased my awareness of the need to adopt a holistic approach to health. A combination of sound medical advice integrated with complementary therapy is, it strikes me, the required formula. This ability to care with humanity is a gift often lacking in modern medicine.

Emma Cannon provides a truly integrated approach to health and well-being based on sound common sense and a human approach to care. This is care in the widest sense of the word. Rather than treating specific conditions, Emma's approach is the general promotion of well-being. Using the framework of Chinese medicine as her starting point, she addresses important factors such as nutrition and lifestyle and understands the importance of the need to take time and space, to nurture and heal and to prevent illness and promote health. In addition, the psychological perspective of self-belief is key. At the same time, there is a clear understanding of the medical issues that can threaten mother and baby requiring good communication with doctors, midwives and other practitioners. In our modern world of more mature mothers who combine career with childbirth, such wisdom is welcome.

Women often tell me how they have been focused on the birth process itself but have lacked advice on preparation for looking after a baby. This continuum is essential and forms another key element in Emma's approach. She has the ability to communicate with the pregnant mother in a non-verbal as well as verbal sense. Working with conventional medical practitioners she has achieved a remarkable synthesis of care. The Health Service is in a state of uncertain flux with challenges of funding. In this environment it is vital not to forget the humanity of care. Emma makes an important contribution to this.

Dr Donald Gibb MD, FRCOG
London, March 2011

introduction

Having a baby . . . is one of the great transitions
we face for which there is no rehearsal. But that
does not mean there can be no preparation.
Naomi Stadlen, What Mothers Do[1]

Whether you have picked up this book as an expectant mother or because you are about to start trying for a baby, I am here to help you help yourself throughout this journey.

You might be focusing on your health for the first time, and it is the perfect time to do so, as your body is amazingly sensitive and intuitive during pregnancy. Most of the time, we crave what is bad for us – salt, sugar, alcohol and the like. But at this time, your body will tend to crave more of what you need, so you can tap into the signs and then carry this through into motherhood and beyond.

Pregnancy is a time when the concepts of cultivating and promoting wellness are likely to make the most sense. You have a new life growing inside you – you are a part of nature's great cycle. Through much of our lives we tend to think of our health only when things go wrong – when we need to find a solution. But when preparing for motherhood we realize that simply *being* healthy can make a positive difference.

When I sat down to start writing this book a phrase popped into my head: 'Let them eat sushi!' You see, I wanted to write a book that moves away from the anxiety about getting everything 'right' during pregnancy and instead empower you with knowledge and choices, allowing you to celebrate your joy and to tap into your instinctive health. As it turns out, you *can* eat sushi but it's one of those little things that are worrying during pregnancy: what can and can't I do? I am interested in helping you to take a positive approach to pregnancy rather than give you a great long list of dos and don'ts.

I am an acupuncturist specializing in pregnancy and fertility, IVF support, postnatal care and gynaecology. Although I studied traditional acupuncture I have always worked with Western medicine, and over the years my treatments have developed into a fusion. I find this fusion works particularly well: my patients feel there is a familiarity about the way I treat them, and they are not overwhelmed by too much new terminology.

My clinic provides an integrated approach to health, combining ortho-dox, Chinese and complementary therapies. With acupuncture underpinning all our treatments we aim to support women through gynaecology, fertility planning, pre-conception, IVF, pregnancy, postnatal and menopausal care. Each patient's personal and individual experience of her health is central to how we diagnose. *Together* we observe where disharmony exists and then work to reinstate balance through a combination of supportive methods.

My first book, *The Baby-Making Bible*, was written out of a heartfelt desire to help couples raise their general health levels prior to conceiving. I did this in the belief and hope that it will improve the health of the children my patients and readers conceive. That theme is continued here, but extends to what you can do once you are pregnant in order to improve the health of your child. And it goes further than health; I believe that a woman's thoughts and deeds during pregnancy can impact on the personality and the entire being of her child.

We spend a long time worrying about room colours and names and fun things like that, but we also need to think about qualities such as kindness and compassion. I want you to consider how the way you think, act and feel could impact on your unborn baby. The Chinese believe that these things greatly affect the developing baby, and there is growing evidence in the West to support this idea. At the very least, pregnancy will give you a chance to prioritize and to think about the importance of these values, both on a personal and a wider community level. I believe babies represent hope; hope in the future that is theirs and ours just for a short time.

This book will help you to:

- ❀ prepare for making a baby, nourishing yourself to create the healthiest environment
- ❀ take care actively of your well-being and that of your unborn child throughout pregnancy
- ❀ fine-tune your health as you encounter some of the common conditions of pregnancy

❀ increase your knowledge of what is going on physiologically and emotionally
❀ prepare your body and mind for birth
❀ prepare for motherhood, supporting you through the first month
❀ enjoy the journey

In Part One, 'Your 360-degree Health Check', you will develop a picture of your general health and well-being. I introduce some simple tools that will help build your body awareness, which is useful throughout pregnancy and into motherhood.

If you are about to start or are currently trying to conceive, Part Two, 'Preparing to Make a Baby', will help you along the way. It's a simple guide through the menstrual cycle, showing how you can optimize your chances of conceiving and where you might need to make tweaks to get your cycle in balance.

Part Three, 'Pregnancy', is split into the three trimesters and is a comprehensive well-being guide to the nine months of pregnancy. I have included my own and other complementary treatments for all the common conditions you might experience, as well as the parallels with Western medicine. I also focus a great deal on preparing during pregnancy, not only for the birth, but also for motherhood, both physically and emotionally.

Part Four, 'Birth', will take you through the stages of labour. It covers acupressure and other pain relievers, positions you can adopt, relaxation exercises and comprehensive information about medical interventions, just in case any are needed.

The six weeks after giving birth to your baby are perhaps the most important in this whole natural process, and in Part Five, 'Postnatal Care', I hope I will inspire you to take this time to nurture your energy to levels that will stay with you through life.

You can read the book from cover to cover, but I also know that many readers will want to dip in and out, and I actively encourage that. Really, this whole book is a preparation for becoming a mother, supporting your health and your emotions and getting you to tap into those wonderful instincts during pregnancy and even before conception. It's easy to see the birth as the end point, whereas of course it's just the beginning.

Blending the Best of East and West: an Integrated Approach

I have one aim with all my patients and that is to optimize their overall health and well-being, creating harmony and balance in the body. It's where I begin with every new patient and so it's the perfect place to start, wherever you are in your baby-making phase or pregnancy.

At the centre of Chinese medicine and its teachings is this idea of balance, and in my mind it extends beyond conception and birth to life in general. By listening to our bodies and our emotions, we can play an important part in our own health. Western medicine has advanced our capabilities to treat problems with amazing speed in the past century, in particular life-threatening conditions, acute illnesses and health crises. If we combine that with traditional Eastern concepts of nurturing our health and our connection with the world around us, then we create an integrated approach that I have found works so effectively with my patients and in my own life.

My interest in women's health really developed when I studied for my acupuncture degree and I was pregnant with my first child. This was a hugely demanding time for me: becoming a mother and studying. Out of necessity, I discovered that both these new challenges in my life nourished and sustained me if I kept them in balance. This experience has formed the basis of my approach to health and has given me great compassion for women who want to become mothers but who also want to retain something of themselves. At the time, I worked at The Gateway clinic in Clapham, London, and there I met an intuitive called Nanette. She told me to focus on bridging the gap between Western and Eastern medicine, that wherever possible I should always work with Western medicine and that Eastern medicine needed straight-thinking people to bring it up to date and to keep it alive.

Her words had a profound impact on me and I knew that what she said was wise and true. To this day, I am always looking for ways to build good working relationships with GPs and specialists and find the common ground. I believe it is what patients want and that working in this way brings optimum beneficial health changes.

The story is told that on Mount Sinai, in addition to the Law, Moses was given a list of all diseases and their cure. This Book was later

destroyed by a pious king who was anxious to restore humility among his subjects. At its best, Western science knows that we can never reconstruct this Book, but it also knows that, in the face of our own incompleteness, we must continue to try. The books of traditional Chinese medicine have been written. The Western book, which is always being created, may yet include Chinese characters.
Ted Kaptchuk, *The Web That Has No Weaver*[2]

I have hung on to this hope for many years, through times when I thought it would not happen. But the fact that I have been asked to write this book, the results that I see with my patients and the growing interest I receive from my colleagues in Western medicine encourage me to believe that some of these valuable and wise theories and treatments will make it into the Western medicine mindset and become part of our treatment protocols. Indeed, it is happening already.

PUTTING MY OWN WORDS INTO PRACTICE

In 2005, I was 37, married to the man I loved and with whom I had my two beautiful children. I thought I was in perfect health and lived the ultimate healthy lifestyle. I was running a successful fertility clinic with highly respected consultant obstetrician Michael Dooley and everything was going from strength to strength.

Suddenly, from nowhere, I was faced with my biggest personal challenge: I was diagnosed with breast cancer. I took the conventional treatment I was offered, which was surgery, chemotherapy and radiotherapy. For me, the radiotherapy was the most aggressive – hot and like fire. Throughout all my treatments, I used my own therapeutic resources to balance the chemicals and the pain. I had acupuncture, put visualization techniques to good use and ate a soothing, cooling diet to counteract the hot aggression of radiotherapy.

Towards the end of the chemotherapy, I experienced some of the most spiritual moments in my life, particularly during my sessions with Emma Roberts, an expert in EFT/meridian tapping who has been kind enough to contribute to this book. It occurred to me that the weaker my body became, the stronger my spirit was. It also reinforced my belief that when one part of the body is weak, something else kicks in and becomes stronger. My daughter Lily's reading advanced five years in ability during that year, clearly her way of coping.

I could not believe how alive I was. My experiences seemed to be super-enhanced – like when you get a new TV and the picture is so much better than the old one. I noticed how much more I was able to help my patients, how direct my treatments had become. No waffle, straight to the point. The conversations that I had with people were deeper and more direct than ever before in my life. People ceased to talk to me about trivial things and began to tell me about their dreams and aspirations.

While I was having my own treatment, I worked a great deal with Emma Roberts on developing my intuition, so that when faced with many options I would instinctively know what to do. Anyone who has been ill, or indeed pregnant, and has been given a great deal of advice by well-meaning relatives and friends (even strangers), will know just how stressful it can be deciding what is important and what is not. It is extremely liberating to discover that you can make choices quickly and without rumination. This skill is something that served me well and helped me with my patients' fertility and pregnancy journeys.

When I was diagnosed, an acupuncture friend of mine said 'lucky you – you will become a master after this'. I laughed, but I have no doubt now that of all my teachers, the year I had cancer and went through treatment was the most profound teacher of all; it was like gaining fifteen years' experience in one. I certainly do not consider myself a master now, but I do consider myself to be lucky.

Chinese medicine

I love the phrase, 'It takes a village to raise a child.' Much of the knowledge I offer has been handed down through generations, from mothers to daughters, practitioners to practitioners. You may instinctively recognize much of the information here, even if Chinese medicine is unfamiliar to you, from the older women in your own family or community, or simply because it feels right and makes sense.

I first discovered Chinese medicine in the mid-1980s (which were all about excess) when I went to see an acupuncturist. I have always been afraid of needles, but I am a big believer in facing your fears, so I decided it was something I needed to overcome. The acupuncturist talked to me for about thirty minutes, she felt my pulse and looked at my tongue (see p. 28). 'Have you suffered from a great grief in your life?' she asked, after considering her findings. I was amazed. 'Yes,' I said. 'My father died when I was sixteen. How did you know?'

She explained to me that in Chinese medicine the Lung is the organ associated with grief and that, from her observations, my Lung Qi (Qi is our energy) was very weak. I did not present with any physical symptoms relating to the lungs from a Western medicine point of view (although I did get a cough every autumn, which is when the lungs are most susceptible), but due to the weakness in my pulse and the crack in the tongue pertaining to the Lung, she had ascertained that the cause must be emotional. She told me she would use points on the Lung meridian to help strengthen the Lung function. She explained it might bring up feelings of grief over the next few weeks.

I lay on the bed, and as soon as she put the needles in I passed out cold! I think she was more alarmed than me, saying this had never happened (it is *very* rare) and that perhaps acupuncture was not the therapy for me. She said I should go away and think it over before booking further treatment.

So that's what I did. Actually, I could think of nothing else. It had been unpleasant passing out and 'losing control' of my body, but from that day something changed. It is difficult to define exactly what it was, but I felt an incredible shift in my emotions and, yes, my energies (I think I was beginning to understand what they were). Far from believing that acupuncture was not the therapy for me, I now thought on the contrary – if it had had such an effect on me, enough for me to pass out and change my feelings, there must be something important to learn from it.

The acupuncturist was right about the grief, which came so gently and full of acceptance. I would be in a supermarket and feel a wave of emotion come over me, tears coming into my eyes and gently rolling down my face. It felt good and full of beauty. I had no idea that acupuncture could help me get in touch with this buried side of me, the young girl who had lost her beloved dad and tried to be brave.

I was drawn to the idea that our physical problems can have their roots in emotional difficulties or that emotional difficulties impact on our physical health. Instinctively, this felt right to me, and I thought that this approach, although thousands of years old, could help many people. Far from feeling old-fashioned, these ideas seemed modern and new to me.

Different patients, different needs

At the heart of Chinese medicine lies diagnosis. It is a complex yet beautifully elegant part of Chinese medicine that I want to tell you about. It teaches us that the same disease or ailment can have many different manifestations and, therefore, require a different treatment. Of course, Chinese medicine diagnosis is far more complex than I will demonstrate in this book, but I hope that I am able to honour it, while at the same time making it accessible. Differential diagnosis is complex and demanding and requires specialized skill on the part of the practitioner. My desire is not to turn you into a practitioner, but to introduce you to some basics that will hopefully raise your self-awareness about your health and develop your intuition. I would encourage you to see a qualified practitioner to deepen your understanding if you want to know more about Chinese medicine.

It saddens me that so many women I see have lost trust in their bodies, usually through over-reliance on the medical profession or through scare stories in the media. There is so much to be gained from understanding your body and the signs it gives you. Not only will this serve you through your pregnancy, but it will help you as a mother to learn about your child and their health. I do believe that wherever possible 'prevention is better than cure' and if you understand your body – how it works and when it goes wrong – you can prevent things from becoming more serious. I am not talking about replacing the doctor here, just being more self-aware.

Preventing things before they become serious is especially true during pregnancy. I find that pregnant women respond extremely well to treatment, and often quickly, if they come as soon as they see the first signs of a condition. If they leave it to become more entrenched, it is often harder to improve things. The same is true for the advice in this book; if you can make small changes quickly, you can help your body to return to normal function. And never put off going to your GP or midwife for serious problems or if symptoms don't clear up quickly.

COMMON CONDITIONS IN PREGNANCY

Throughout the book, you will find some of the major and common conditions of pregnancy. Each condition is set out with differential diagnosis where relevant; in other words, the different ways in which it can manifest. You will be asked to consider some details about a condition in a way that may be new to you. In the case of morning sickness, for example, I will ask you if you feel like you can't get out of bed, or if you feel chilly or hot. Each manifestation of morning sickness will require a slightly different treatment; you will discover that not all morning sickness responds well to using ginger and why some morning sickness does not happen in the morning. There will also be ideas and tips on how best to treat the condition.

I have also asked some of my complementary therapy colleagues to contribute their tips to help you, from osteopathy to reflexology and yoga. And in the Resources section (see p. 339), you will find useful numbers of various associations to help you find local practitioners.

An Introduction to the Therapies

I thought it was important to try and write this book in a way that is as close as possible to the way I work in my practice. That means working in collaboration. And so throughout the book you will come across information and tips from other healthcare practitioners. I am often known to pick up the phone to a colleague mid-consultation and ask, 'What do you think of X or Y?' I am never afraid to ask others' opinions and have talked about health ideas for many years with colleagues; of course, we don't always agree, but there is dialogue and that is what matters. My experience is that patients want the best of both worlds; they don't mind what they have to do (within reason), as long as it works.

I have worked for many years in collaboration with some of the finest practitioners in the country – both from Western and complementary medicine. I work with people who have open minds, people who know that their medicine is not the only medicine, and together we are able to offer our patients options, empowering them to make informed decisions.

So I have brought together here a team of health providers who have each made invaluable contributions to the book – my 'village'. Now I am not suggesting that we'll need the cast of *Ben Hur* to support you through pregnancy, only that I have picked some of the best brains in the country to order to give you ideas to explore and try for yourself.

Every pregnancy is individual, every journey different. There is no magic wand, no one-size-fits-all, but any journey you take (good or bad) helps you to discover new things, skills you did not know you had. Maybe nature meant for us to learn some life lessons during pregnancy; you will certainly learn patience, which will come in handy later as a parent. *Your* pregnancy is *your* journey – an exciting ride of discovery. It is a precious time and I hope we can help you enjoy it.

Midwifery

Your midwife (or midwife team) is there as a helping hand through your pregnancy and labour, often picking up conditions very early on or preventing them. It's very important to feel comfortable with your midwife and the team, and if you are lucky enough to see the same midwife throughout your pregnancy and birth, this can be of great emotional and practical comfort. If you are unable to meet the actual person (or persons) who will be your midwife through labour then it will be helpful to have someone you can rely on to be there as a support for you throughout the birth as well as your partner, perhaps a female friend or relative.

Anna Cannon is a midwife with over twenty years' experience, and also happens to be my sister-in-law. Anna has very kindly contributed to Parts Four and Five in the book and offers invaluable advice for you to carry with you through your pregnancy and the first weeks and months of becoming a mum. In her words:

> As midwives we are complementary to nature. Our primary role is to encourage women's natural abilities to have children, to empower you with informed choices and build your confidence as a mother. Throughout the journey of pregnancy the midwife has an advocacy role, and especially during birth we are your advocate at a time when you can't think straight.

Obstetrics

Many consultants practise both obstetrics and gynaecology. Consultant obstetricians play an essential role in the care of pregnant women who are at a higher risk of certain conditions or complications – for example, if you are having multiples, are an older woman or have had previous pregnancy problems or conditions that might impact on pregnancy. The obstetrician is there to keep an eye on things throughout pregnancy and labour when things are out of the ordinary. Usually, if you need to see an obstetrician there will also be more tests and close monitoring involved, all for your own and your baby's health and well-being.

Acupuncture

For many people who have tried acupuncture treatment for chronic pain it can only be described as magic. It certainly isn't easy to explain how a tiny needle you can hardly feel might have such a dramatic effect. But it goes back to the concept at the heart of Chinese medicine: that of creating balance and harmony in the body for health and well-being.

Our Qi courses through our bodies continuously, making connections and activating channels of energy. There are acupuncture points on the surface of our skin that are best described as gateways into this network or Qi. When, as a specialist, I insert the acupuncture needles at these points, I do so to either activate or inhibit the flow of energy there. Over many generations, we have learnt which combinations of points do what, and with this knowledge we can treat a whole array of conditions.

Acupuncture has become particularly well known for pain relief and in the field of fertility. There is a growing body of scientific evidence to support the anecdotal claims associated with this treatment.[3]

Acupressure

When I first became interested in complementary therapies I studied and practised Shiatsu. Shiatsu is similar to acupuncture in theory, but instead of using needles, the practitioner applies pressure to the points and channels, using thumbs, elbows, forearms or sometimes even knees. It is a wonderful feeling and, because of the close contact between practitioner and patient, it feels very supportive.

Acupressure is a simplified version of Shiatsu. It is easy to practise yourself or for your partner to use on you. During or prior to labour, it is a lovely way to involve your partner and give him something helpful to do for you. I have included easy-to-follow acupressure techniques in this book so that you can practise at home. I recommend using mainly thumbs to apply pressure (although we may improvise sometimes). Throughout the book, I have suggested acupuncture points that I would use for certain conditions; I have only given you the main points and the ones that tend to function well even when used in isolation. The idea is to apply pressure to these points – fixed pressure is best (although some people prefer to use small circular movements). This is not massage, and sometimes it can feel uncomfortable to apply strong pressure to these points. But if the pressure is applied gradually and evenly, you should be able to tolerate it and feel the brilliant benefits. I have included diagrams with instructions showing where acupressure is particularly beneficial. You can also use ear-press seeds – minute seeds or grains that can be placed on the points and kept in place with plasters (see Resources).

Yoga

Yoga is an excellent way to connect to your body and the changes it goes through during pregnancy, and also to help manage those changes. It's extremely good for stress relief and, through being so aware of and focused on your breath and the body positions, yoga literally takes you out of your head and calms the mind. It's the perfect antidote to modern living, and also gives you a wonderful sense of body confidence, helping you to understand your body's abilities and power during this amazing transformation.

Throughout the book, there are key introductory yoga principles and poses – these have been generously provided by Uma Dinsmore-Tuli (see Resources, p. 344, and Further Reading, p. 347, for a full list of Uma's books and contact details). Uma describes yoga as a complete system of self-care and spiritual growth that promotes well-being and a positive experience throughout pregnancy. During pregnancy the best approach is to keep yoga simple and effective, using it to promote three crucial aspects of health and well-being: the way you *breathe*, how you *move* and your capacity to *rest and be*. With these three elements working together throughout the three trimesters, yoga can help you breathe fully to enhance your vitality, move freely and gracefully and enable you to rest completely, so that you can enjoy each moment as it comes. There are also yoga techniques for labour and postnatal care and recovery.

Meridian tapping (EFT)

Meridian tapping is also derived from acupuncture and is a way to free ourselves from the ongoing emotional and physical damage caused by traumas we have experienced. It involves gentle tapping of the same energy points as acupuncture, while at the same time focusing on the specific emotional issue to clear energy blockages that might be obstructing our efforts to achieve our goals.

Emma Roberts is a pioneer of EFT (Emotional Freedom Techniques) and meridian tapping in the UK and has contributed tapping exercises here for significant emotional issues often linked with fertility, pregnancy and motherhood. (See p. 35 for an overview of how to get started with tapping.)

Reflexology

Reflexology is very helpful for the tired and heavy-leg feeling many women experience during pregnancy. It is not based on the same system as Chinese medicine, and there is a debate as to whether it originated in Egypt, India, China or even South America. I find it to be very relaxing and balancing, and it is especially good for patients who really cannot get on with needles. Many pregnant women also tend to forget that there is anything below their bump; reflexology brings the focus and energy down from the head throughout the body to the tips of the hands and feet.

Although foot reflexology is commonly known, people aren't so familiar with hand reflexology. The theory of reflexology is that organs, nerves, glands and parts of the body are connected to reflex areas or points on both the feet and hands. By stimulating these areas, a direct response can be created in the related body area.

This stimulation releases blocked energy pathways and therefore enables the body to heal. One of the main benefits of hand reflexology during pregnancy (after the first trimester) is that it is a safe, natural, empowering healing that you can use yourself with amazing results. It can help to relieve a long list of pregnancy-associated symptoms, from nausea, to constipation, through to carpal-tunnel syndrome and sinusitis. Reflexology can be administered anywhere and at any time, as and when needed. (See p. 334 for the basic techniques.)

Note: Reflexology is safe throughout pregnancy, although it should only be administered after the first thirteen weeks to allow the body to settle. Pregnancy conditions and circumstances where reflexology is contraindicated include a history of miscarriage, pre-term labour and, if you are thirty-two weeks or more into pregnancy, placenta praevia (low-lying placenta) and hydroamnios (excess amniotic fluid around the baby). If in any doubt, speak to your consultant before treatment.

Osteopathy

During pregnancy your body needs to adapt to carrying your growing baby, changing your relationship to gravity. Osteopathy is a holistic therapy that aims to keep your body in good structural balance. It can identify stresses and strains related to your history and recognize postural compensations. Osteopathy uses a wide range of gentle manipulation techniques and includes massage, cranial treatment and joint mobilization. In the pregnancy section I have included tips from an osteopath on posture, sleep positions and how to adapt to your growing bump.

Moxibustion and warming techniques

These are the techniques used to warm the body in the case of Cold, Cold/ Damp and Yang Deficient (which I'll explain on p. 39), especially when the lower abdomen is cold to touch.

In moxibustion, a herbal stick (moxa) is lit and held over acupuncture points or other areas of the body in order to warm and activate them (see p. 333). I also give patients a 'Womb Warmer' to use at home; this is a small heat pad that can be placed on the lower abdomen and used again and again. Moxibustion is something that is easy and safe to do at home, but I recommend that you see a qualified acupuncturist for an introductory session to familiarize yourself with the treatment (see Resources, p. 339).

Aromatherapy

Aromatherapy is the use of essential oils as a natural remedy. The oils are diluted in a base oil (almond, for example) and can be burnt, used in the bath or for massage. I have included remedies for later pregnancy, preparing for birth and for post-natal recovery.

Note: Some oils are best avoided during pregnancy, and all essential oils should be avoided in the first trimester. This isn't because aromatherapy is dangerous, but there isn't sufficient research into their safety, so the advice is a precaution. Neals Yard Remedies is extremely helpful for checking the use of any essential oils (see Resources, p. 342).

Chinese Medicine Explained

Differential diagnosis lies at the heart of Chinese medicine. We look at the body and mind as a whole, using symptoms as signals for discovering under-lying imbalances. The language may sound rather strange and unfamiliar at first, but my hope is that it soon begins to feel like common sense, especially as you tap in to your own body awareness.

The following is an introduction to the main terms I use in the book. Whenever I refer to a Chinese medicine term, I give it a capital letter (Qi or Liver, for example). This is because Liver in Chinese medicine has a far wider meaning than that attributed to the word in Western terms. Chinese medicine ascribes not only function, but also emotional features to organs: the Liver, for instance, is associated with the drive for life, vision and is also connected to the eyes. So when you see a capital letter in the text, we are talking Chinese medicine. As you read through the book, the terms will become increasingly familiar, and I hope you will see just how far they are steeped in logic.

Qi

Qi, pronounced 'chee', is at the very heart of Chinese medicine. Qi is our life force; it is that unquantifiable energy that runs through our bodies and which makes us grow and learn and function as human beings.

Healthy Qi is like a fresh, cool breeze. It flows easily. Unhealthy Qi is like an oppressive, thundery day where the air feels heavy and stuck. Much of Chinese medicine is concerned with keeping the Qi flowing with strength and continuity. The twelve meridians are the pathways along which Qi flows through the body, and acupuncture points are found along those merid-ians, acting as gateways for blocking or unblocking it. Massage is designed to improve the flow of energy through touch, while aromatherapy opens up the channels through our sense of smell. All of these therapies encourage the body's own healing processes, whether physical, mental or emotional.

Yin and Yang

Yin and Yang are again central to the importance of balance and of the cycles of nature within Chinese medicine. The iconic 'Yin Yang' symbol represents the two opposing yet interdependent energies. Yin is cool, nourishing and calming, associated with the feminine, whereas Yang, associated with the masculine, is active, motivating and warm.

When healthy, Yin and Yang are in harmony, and it is our ability to adapt and fine-tune when faced with changing conditions that maintains our balance. During menstruation, Yin represents the beginning part of your cycle and Yang takes over in the second phase, when you become a human incubator for the fertilized egg. In conception the Yin is the egg (the hold potential) and the Yang is the sperm (the activator). In pregnancy, Yin dominates as, again, it is a time of beginning, while Yang dominates for birth – as it is a time for active energy.

The simple therapies and nutrition I recommend for preparing to conceive, for pregnancy and getting ready for birth and early motherhood are all closely linked to creating a healthy balance, depending on the energy you need.

Jing

A fundamental principle of Chinese medicine is that your health is affected by that of your parents. This is your ancestral health. There is prenatal Jing and postnatal Jing; once you are born you can't change your prenatal Jing, but you can affect your postnatal Jing through your environment and lifestyle and can, therefore, pass on good Jing to your own children (just as in Western medicine we talk of health predispositions signposted in our genes, but we also know there is much we can do ourselves to affect our health).

In Chapter Two (see p. 32) you can gauge your own Jing and find out how to pass good Jing down through the generations.

The Five Climates

The Five Climates are linked to nature and the seasonal climates. In Chinese medicine we use these terms to describe a patient's internal climate. You may tend towards a particular type or show signs of a combination, depending on the 'current conditions'. I will refer to these Climates throughout the book, as they are an excellent way to detect how you are feeling and how you can make small adjustments, like adding a certain food or tea to your diet to bring you back into healthy balance.

Cold

Just as in winter, cold slows things down. It is constricting and can depress the body's natural functions – for example, the digestion and immune system. Cold is often accompanied by a lack of energy and feelings of weariness.

Heat

Heat is essential for energy, but in excess it can cause inflammation and fever. This heat will often rise to the surface through a reddish appearance, increased perspiration and skin conditions. Internally, heat is often signalled by thirst, constipation and feeling agitated.

Damp

Damp is the term used to describe an overly moist or wet condition, where fluids have accumulated inappropriately. Damp has a sluggish, stagnant, heavy feel. Water retention, bloating, excess weight, fatigue, lack of appetite and a heavy feeling are all signs of excess Damp.

Dry

Brittle hair and nails, dry skin conditions and constipation are all associated with dryness in the body. These are signs of dehydration, when body fluids are lost or damaged, often by Heat.

Wind

Just as an 'ill wind blows', in Chinese medicine Wind is considered a strong force for upsetting the balance. External Wind that invades the body often manifests as a cold or flu, sometimes bringing with it Damp, Cold, Dryness or Heat in the form of phlegm, shivers, a dry tickly throat or fever. Signs of internal Wind include headaches, tremors, seizures and emotional instability.

Blood

Blood is extremely important in Chinese medicine. Blood transports vitality, the Qi. As many as 60 per cent of the women I see have an element of Blood Deficiency. It doesn't necessarily mean you are anaemic (see p. 134 for anaemia in pregnancy), but you might be on the road to iron deficiency.

Phlegm

Phlegm is a result of excess Damp, and many pregnant women are prone to conditions that bring excess phlegm and mucus with them. Often, Phlegm is a sign of digestive weakness, particularly associated with the Spleen.

Stagnation

There are two types of Stagnation: Qi and Blood. Qi Stagnation is something we all suffer from at some point in our life. It is signalled by sudden flares in temper, being prone to high emotions and indecision. Left untreated, it often turns into Heat (see p. 17). Blood Stagnation is where your blood doesn't move around the body as freely as it should. It is linked closely to Qi Stagnation and often presents itself as broken veins under the skin, varicose veins, fibroids or endometriosis.

'Deficient'

You might be Yin Deficient or Yang Deficient, leading to an imbalance of these opposite yet interdependent energies. Yin Deficiency (see p. 38) usually occurs in patients with severe Heat or in those who are seriously Blood Deficient. The symptoms of Yang Deficiency (see p. 39) are linked to those of Cold, but more extreme.

'Excess'

'Excess' is related to the Five Climates. We look, therefore, both for signs of deficiency and excess and then seek to make adjustments to help rebalance the body's natural health. Excess requires that we clear a climate from the body, so as to regain equilibrium – for example too much Damp or Cold will need to be cleared to balance things out again.

The Organs

From a Chinese Medicine viewpoint everything is interconnected – no part of the body stands alone and each organ has an emotion attributed to it. All the organs are connected by internal pathways known as channels, within which flows the all-important Qi.

Kidneys

The Kidneys are the Water element of the body – one of their functions being to excrete impure fluids from the body. The Water element represents the season of winter and the source of all life – it is the foundation of life and reproduction. It is said that the Kidneys house and store the Jing (Jing being responsible for birth, reproduction, growth and all human development). The stronger the Jing, the healthier and more fertile the person. Jing is what we pass on to our children – it could be understood as our genetic blueprint or our constitution.

Our sexuality is rooted in Kidney energy, including our ability to engage in a healthy, loving sex life free from guilt and shame. From that Jing your body also produces marrow which fills up the bones and makes them strong. The teeth and hair too come from this same source. The Kidneys make their connection to the outside world through the ears. A person's ability to hear clearly is reflected in the strength of their Kidneys.

On an emotional level, the Kidneys represent our drive for life, our will-power and our ability to pass on this will to the next generation. When the Kidneys are weak, we have weak will and easily give into fear and paranoia.

Liver and Gall Bladder

The Liver and the Gall Bladder represent the Wood element and also the season of spring.

The Liver makes sure that Qi flows smoothly and gets to every part of the body that needs it. When this is effective, all our bodily functions work smoothly and we feel relaxed and easy-going. When the Qi is thwarted on its journey, it becomes stagnant and stuck and we feel frustrated and depressed. The Liver is connected to us realizing our potential in life. With a strong Liver energy, we overcome life's difficulties with ease and determination. When we don't, anger and frustration ensue. The Liver gives us our drive, vision and direction in life and makes its connection to the outside world through the eyes.

The Gall Bladder supports the Liver and plays an important role in decision-making and initiative. On a physical level, it stores and excretes bile from the body and helps the Liver regulate Qi.

Heart

The Fire element is the Heart, representing summer. In Chinese medicine the Heart is connected to the Shen, the mind. When the Heart and the Blood are strong, the Shen is settled and the emotional life is well balanced. When they are out of balance, we may suffer from anxiety and nervousness.

The Heart is the supreme ruler, and it is important that it remains settled and calm. In pregnancy, it has an important role through its strong connection with the uterus. During pregnancy, your baby is nourished emotionally through this internal connection. The Heart also represents communication and therefore connects to the world and with others through speech and singing.

Spleen and Stomach

Earth is the next element, representing late summer and the organs Spleen and Stomach. These organs play the vital role of digestion from which the body makes Qi and Blood. They take in and give out nourishment. They like to be warm, and they give the muscles strength and form. The qualities of the Earth element are those of the archetypal mother.

On an emotional level, the Spleen and Stomach represent how good we are at nourishing ourselves, which is vital for mothers to learn. Learning to nourish ourselves, both emotionally and through nutrition, is a central theme in pregnancy. The Spleen governs the body's ability to think, concentrate and to absorb ideas. When weak, there is a tendency to be self-absorbed and overly concerned for oneself. Worry and rumination occur when the Earth element is weak; when it is strong the thought process is clear and focused.

Lungs

Finally, we come to the Metal element, representing autumn and governed by the Lung and Large Intestine. Metal represents the father, our self-values, beliefs and ability to become our own person as we grow up.

The Lung takes in Qi from the air that you breathe and circulates it to the whole body. Breath is so important in pregnancy and childbirth. In childbirth, it is said that part of the mother's soul that presides in the Lung enters the baby and can be heard through its first cry. The mother's breath is vital in pregnancy and can strongly impact on the strength of her contractions.

So the Lungs take in usable Qi from the air you breathe and the Large Intestine lets go of Qi in its unusable form. Weakness in this element is associated with an inability to take in and let go of things on an emotional level, so you can see how important this function is during childbirth. It is vital to be able to take in a breath and then to let go in order to help move the baby down inside the birth canal.

These are some of the core building blocks in Chinese medicine, and I hope that they are already beginning to feel familiar to you, even if the terminology takes a little getting used to. In the next chapter, we begin to build on those foundation blocks with 'Your 360-degree Health Check' – a whole-body MOT.

part one

YOUR 360-DEGREE HEALTH CHECK

Whenever I meet a new patient, I encourage them to slow down and take time to look at their health and well-being in the whole, hence the 360-degree health check. Whether you are preparing to make a baby or already have, this is the perfect time to spring clean your diet and lifestyle gently – it is a time of beginning, and so starting afresh is helpful both for your body and mind in preparation for the months ahead.

This is certainly not a time for guilt or feeling anxious that you might be getting things wrong. Taking care of your health and sense of well-being is the biggest gift and it's not about rights or wrongs. It's finding *your* balance that matters.

I break down the 360-degree check into three areas:

1. Is the engine working?

I define 'the engine' as your physical health, the development and health of your baby during pregnancy and into the first month after birth, and the lifestyle and environmental factors that may have an impact.

2. Is the fuel good?

The fuel is what you put into your body, both for you and your baby. Placing importance on diet and good digestion is vital.

3. Is the mind on board?

Your mind plays a key role in your health and well-being, and that of your baby. Dealing with stress effectively during pregnancy and understanding the links between your emotions and health are extremely helpful over the next few months and beyond into motherhood.

These three areas are not separate, but interconnected and each is involved in the function of the others. Everything in Chinese medicine exists as part of a whole problem and nothing is ever treated in isolation. Your body, mind and environment are inseparable, and each has influence on the other.

Some readers will automatically be attracted to one approach or another. But that does not necessarily mean that this is where they need the most work. If someone eats really well, but never rests, and their digestion is poor and they work in, say, a hostile environment, then all that good diet will achieve is damage limitation. Someone who has a weak Spleen function may become rather self-absorbed and obsessive about diet, monitoring everything they put into their body. More dietary advice may not, therefore, be the right approach for them. Perhaps they need to be more outward looking and less controlling over food.

As you read the book, ask yourself, 'Is it my engine, the fuel or my mind?' and address some of the areas where your natural response would be, 'This doesn't apply to me.' Take a second look; there is often a great deal to learn when we face our fears, and if you feel daft saying positive things about yourself, then maybe that's a good thing – maybe you will soften towards yourself by doing it. The key is that *you* decide.

chapter one
DEVELOPING SELF-AWARENESS

I am going to talk you through the process of diagnosis in Chinese medicine, which when I first started learning acupuncture made sense to me like nothing ever had before. It described a way of viewing the world and health that resonated deeply with me – I was hooked.

It is a different approach to looking at symptoms; if a patient comes to me with one specific symptom, I want to know how that symptom fits into their health in general. I am not focused on the cause of that one symptom, but on how it appeared as a part of the whole. So instead of asking, 'How did X cause Y?', I'll consider, 'What is the relationship between X and Y?'

As you read through the following section, I'd encourage you to make your own notes. Keeping a journal throughout your pregnancy (and even pre-conception) can help you to reflect on how you are feeling physically and emotionally, and keep reminders for those things you try that work well, or not. It's also useful to remember that your body and environment are constantly adjusting, even slightly, and so while you might strongly recognize some of the symptoms below, the picture will alter over time. So it's helpful to check back and see how your fine-tuning is improving your general sense of well-being. With this will come self-awareness and you will begin to feel confident that you have some input into your own health, developing your personal responsibility.

How Is Your Qi?

If you jump out of bed in the morning full of energy and ready for the day ahead then you likely have great Qi. If, on the other hand, you hit the snooze button six times before dragging yourself out of bed, and can't speak a civil word before your first cup of tea, it's likely that your Qi is depleted.

Your Qi will be evident in your:

- ❁ overall energy
- ❁ demeanour
- ❁ voice
- ❁ complexion.

Here are some questions to ask yourself:

- ❁ Do I get ill often?
- ❁ Am I frequently tired?
- ❁ Do I find it hard to recover from illness?
- ❁ Am I the first to leave a party?
- ❁ Do I find it hard to get out of bed in the morning?
- ❁ Do I have a 'quiet' or 'thin' voice?
- ❁ Does my skin look tired?

If you answer 'Yes' to more than four of the above, you are exhibiting some tell-tale signs of depleted Qi – a sort of less-than-best vitality. I see many pregnant women who have signs of Qi Stagnation, probably because their energy is in such great demand. It often manifests as indigestion and gas, or in the mood as feelings of frustration or sighing.

How can you cultivate good Qi?

Take a gentle approach to building up your Qi. Avoid making any radical, sudden changes; begin by looking at these areas:

- ❁ Eat well.
- ❁ Balance your emotions and resolve conflicts.
- ❁ Understand your constitutional strengths and weaknesses – your Jing (see p. 43).
- ❁ Don't compare yourself to others.
- ❁ Balance your working life (see p. 32).

❀ Keep the engine well oiled – gentle walking, yoga and qigong (a form of exercise designed to build and improve the movement of Qi) all help to generate Qi within the body.

Your Menstrual Cycle

It is said that a good practitioner of Chinese medicine can tell everything about a woman's health from her menstrual symptoms alone. The hormones that facilitate the cycle, like a wheel kept in motion by water, determine your mood, the way you look, feel, behave and even the way you dress.

If you are trying to conceive, Part Two, 'Preparing to Make a Baby', takes you through the twenty-eight-day cycle and can help you look at whether there are simple measures you can take to help create the perfect balance.

Your Eyes

The eyes are important for diagnosis in both Western and Chinese medicine. They reveal the health of the liver and emotions in particular. Eyes betray tiredness, a night out, sadness and hurt; they also sparkle when full of joy.

Ideally, your eyes are clear and bright, full of vitality. Look in the mirror and see if they match any of these descriptions:

❀ Cloudy – may indicate an unsettled mind and Qi Stagnation.
❀ Dull – may indicate an emotional issue that needs to be addressed.
❀ Red – can indicate Heat and tiredness.
❀ Yellowing in the whites – shows ill health and Qi Deficiency.
❀ Puffy – this can be caused by Dampness.
❀ Dark rings – a well-recognized sign that you are not getting enough sleep. It can also signify reproductive weakness and Kidney weakness.
❀ Weeping or watery – you may literally be grieving or sad and show tears you are unable to cry.
❀ Red, weeping and watery – can be hay fever, which is sometimes a symptom of Damp.
❀ Bloodshot – can indicate suppressed anger.

Your Mouth and Lips

Chinese medicine makes a connection between the health of the digestive system and the appearance of the mouth and lips. Problems here can reveal digestive disturbance and the clues to how we are nourishing ourselves.

Colour of lips

The normal colour and condition of lips is pale red, moist and slightly shiny. Have a look to see if yours match any of the following descriptions:

- ❀ Pale with a blueish or purple tinge – Cold.
- ❀ Very red – Heat.
- ❀ Pale and dry – Blood Deficient.
- ❀ Cracked at the corners – this can indicate a Vitamin B deficiency, and a supplement (such as folic acid, which is key for conception and pregnancy) should be taken.
- ❀ Greenish in hue – Qi Stagnation.
- ❀ Swollen – indicates problems with the digestive system; Damp.
- ❀ Cold sores – can point to localized Damp Heat.
- ❀ Spots on the chin – may indicate Blood Stagnation.

Your Tongue

The tongue is one of the most famous diagnostic tools in Chinese medicine, giving up a great deal of information about your health. As a practitioner, I have great tomes that chart even minuscule differences in the condition of the tongue. Patients nearly fall off their chairs when I look at their tongues and ask pertinent questions based on what I see. Here are the broad categories so you can begin to see for yourself what your tongue says about your health:

Colour, coat and texture

The ideal tongue colour is pale red. It should be slightly wet, with no significant marks. Colour variations may include:

- ❀ red – Heat
- ❀ purple – Stagnation

- ❀ pale – Blood Deficiency
- ❀ orange sides – Blood Deficiency
- ❀ red tip – Heat in the Heart (indicating anxiety, often with disturbed sleep)
- ❀ blue – Cold/Stagnation.

As for variations in coat/texture, these may include:

- ❀ heavily coated – a sign of poor digestive function and Dampness; the patient will usually be a little sluggish and may feel general malaise
- ❀ dirty brown or thick and yellow coating – may indicate Damp/Heat
- ❀ white and thick coating – shows a tendency towards Cold/Damp
- ❀ cracked along the centre – may indicate Yin Deficiency or Heat (if it reaches the end it's Heart weakness)
- ❀ teeth marks – can indicate poor digestive function
- ❀ involuntary quivering – indicates Qi Deficiency.

Your Skin

The skin, the largest organ of the human body, reveals a lot about a person's health. It is said to be the 'third lung' and this connection is seen in the close relationship between asthma and its outward manifestation eczema. Here are some signs to look out for:

- ❀ Redness – Heat
- ❀ A very oily complexion – Damp
- ❀ Weeping sores – Damp Heat
- ❀ Itchy skin – Blood Deficient
- ❀ Noticeable pallor – often means Blood Deficient
- ❀ Dry Skin – Blood Deficient
- ❀ Puffy skin that leaves an indent – Dampness and fluid retention
- ❀ Breakouts on the chin – can indicate Stagnation and/or Damp Heat in the reproductive system

- ❀ Yellow tinge – suggests problems with the liver
- ❀ Green tinge – Stagnation
- ❀ Black tinge – localized congestion, Blood Stagnation

Excessive sweating can be indicative of Heat (especially if you are throwing off the covers at night), Yin Deficiency (an advanced state of Heat) or Dampness.

Your Urine

A healthy, well-hydrated person goes to the loo around five to seven times a day. Ideally, your urine should be clear and very slightly yellow. Problems with urine usually involve the Kidney/Bladder energy:

- ❀ Cloudy – Dampness
- ❀ Very frequent – weak Qi
- ❀ Plentiful and clear – Cold
- ❀ Dark and scanty – Heat (and dehydration)
- ❀ Dribbling after urination – indicates weak Qi

Your Stools

Yes, we scrutinize everything in Chinese medicine. Ideally, we would all pass perfectly formed stools shortly after rising in the morning. However, these are all possibilities:

- ❀ Constipation, followed by small, bitty stools ('rabbit droppings') – Qi Stagnation
- ❀ Constipation with pain and a cold tummy – Cold or Damp/Cold
- ❀ Constipation where the stool is dry – Blood Deficient or Heat
- ❀ Constipation followed by diarrhoea (typical of IBS) – Qi Stagnation
- ❀ Strong-smelling stools – Damp/Heat
- ❀ Mucus in stools – Damp
- ❀ Black or dark stools – Blood Stagnation
- ❀ Wind – normally indicates Qi Stagnation
- ❀ Wind with strong smell – Damp/Heat

HELPING WITH COLD TENDENCIES

Do	Don't
Drink teas, such as ginger tea	Eat food straight from the
Eat warming foods (see p. 39)	fridge
Eat mainly cooked food	Drink ice-cold liquids
Take warming baths	Eat raw foods
Sleep away from the window and draughts	Walk on stone floors with
Keep your midriff warm at all times	bare feet

HELPING WITH HEAT TENDENCIES

Do	Don't
Eat cooling and neutral foods (see p. 59)	Drink alcohol or caffeine
Practice meditation and yoga for calming	Eat chocolate, greasy foods
Manage your stress	or sugar
	Eat heating foods (see p. 58)

HELPING WITH DAMP TENDENCIES

Do	Don't
Eat fresh foods	Drink alcohol
Drink barley water (see p. 215)	Eat dairy foods, chocolate,
Drink jasmine tea, green tea, fennel tea	curries, bread, wheat, fried
Eat Damp-resolving foods (see p. 58)	foods or sugar
	Eat late at night
	Eat proteins and
	carbohydrates together

By now, you will have begun to compile a list of symptoms; perhaps you have identified some Cold symptoms or Qi Deficiency. Keep these to hand as you read the next few chapters, 'Is the Engine Working?', 'Is the Fuel Good?' and 'Is the Mind on Board?' You may start to recognize areas where your health might be out of balance, and see how you can start to implement small lifestyle changes. Remember, your health isn't set in stone, so as you develop your awareness you'll be able to adjust and fine-tune your diet and lifestyle to suit.

chapter two
IS THE ENGINE WORKING?

Is your body in top condition with everything running smoothly? Think about the areas in your life or environment where you might need a little more balance.

Work Life Balance

We live in a society that places a great deal of importance on overwork and overachieving. Illness and feeling tired are seen as an inconvenience that gets in the way. Many women work in desk jobs, sitting at the computer all day with poor posture, staring at a bright screen for hours on end, not going out, even for a lunchtime walk and some fresh air. Making endless cups of tea and coffee provides the only chance for a quick break, so becomes habitual.

Whatever your workplace, it's easy to fall into the trap of working long hours and living on stress. It's often how we get ahead in today's economy. If we want to succeed and be high achievers, we have to put in the extra hours and effort – life can come later. It is not surprising that we exhaust our Qi, or that diseases which Chinese medicine describes as those of 'excess' are more common in Western cultures.

Think about how much time you spend on work and your commute. If you leave home at 7 a.m. and arrive back in the evening at 9 p.m. you are spending fourteen hours of your day on work, seven to eight hours sleeping and that leaves three hours for your life. When your baby arrives, you will be making massive adjustments, so it's worth thinking about this potential imbalance now at this early stage.

Can you start looking at ways to make space for a baby? It's not about giving up your job or your ambitions, but can you be a little smarter with your time? If your employers support flexible working hours, can you give them a test run? Perhaps with some creative thinking your job could be done in fewer than five days a week. And try working smarter in less time – it's amazing what you can get done when you have to be at the nursery by a set time; if you can start practising now, the benefits to your general health at this early stage will be immense.

If you are extremely hardworking, you might be what we call Blood Deficient in Chinese medicine, sometimes associated with anaemia in pregnancy (see p. 134).

Here are some ways to deal with early tendencies towards Blood Deficiency, which are good advice for all:

- ❀ Eat regular meals in a relaxed environment.
- ❀ Don't stay up late to work – get a good night's sleep and relax before you go to bed.
- ❀ Include nourishing soups in your diet (see recipes for chicken soup, p. 314, and sweet potato and lentil soup, p. 179).
- ❀ Include foods to nourish the Blood (see chart, p. 57).
- ❀ Avoid alcohol (or have occasionally with food).
- ❀ Try not to push yourself beyond your limits.
- ❀ Take your holiday.
- ❀ Exercise in the morning, rather than at the end of the day.

Underactive

While some women work all hours in the competition to get ahead, many who are at the other end of the scale may find their work boring, or perhaps unfulfilling.

Being unfulfilled impacts on your health and your whole way of being, and one word in Chinese medicine sums it up perfectly: Stagnation.

If you are preparing to make a baby, dealing with Stagnation will help to get your Qi moving and literally put you in the right frame of mind for conceiving. And even if you are thrilled at having become pregnant, it's a great idea to tackle Stagnation if you recognize the signs when it comes to work. Becoming a parent really does put life into perspective, so you can use that now to think about the future and how to make sure you don't get stuck in any ruts:

- ❀ Spend time thinking about the question, 'What is my purpose in life?' Write down your thoughts and make a plan.
- ❀ Bring creativity into your life – through hobbies, cooking, culture.
- ❀ Keep a 'gratitude diary' – find something each day to give thanks for.
- ❀ Replace complaining with an active search for solutions – take responsibility.

Stress

Even the word 'stress' conjures up the feelings we all experience at times. While a little stress is, in fact, good for us, it's all a matter of balance. Too much stress and, even more importantly, how we deal with it, has been shown to be clearly harmful to our health.

When we are in a stressful situation, our body's natural defence modes kick in and we adopt our ancient 'fight-or-flight' response. This causes our adrenal glands to secrete cortisol (the stress hormone) and adrenalin into the bloodstream to give us the burst of energy and strength needed either to fight (the woolly mammoth) or for flight (run like crazy). In the situations that usually trigger stress in our modern lives, we rarely need either response, so that if we don't know how to relax, we can find ourselves living in a permanent state of stress with far too much cortisol building up in our bodies.

When you are preparing to make a baby, stress can ruin your sex life and even prevent your body from releasing an egg; while in pregnancy, stress can aggravate nausea. A relaxed mum has been shown to benefit the health of her unborn child – calm mum equals calm baby.

We have many constraints on us in life, and this can stifle our free-flowing nature. When this happens, we say that Qi is Stagnant, and from this anger and frustration can result.

And relax . . .

Learning how to relax is an essential tool for life and for parenthood. Your baby will trigger a stress response in you every time she cries and you can't work out why. Your toddler will raise your stress levels with every supermarket tantrum. If you can teach yourself how to relax when faced with challenging situations, the benefits will extend beyond just your health. You'll find yourself a more confident parent and your toddler will soon see that tantrums don't lead to the heights of attention they were hoping for.

Tools for relaxation
❀ Yoga and qigong (see p. 41)
❀ Meditation (see p. 64)
❀ Meridian tapping (see below)

FOOD TIP

Calming foods include celery, chamomile and lettuce.
Foods to raise the spirits include basil, jasmine, oats, rosemary and sage.

Meridian tapping

Meridian tapping (also known as Emotional Freedom Techniques or EFT, the name given to meridian tapping by Gary Craig, the American founder[4]) uses the same energy points as acupuncture. Gentle tapping of these points, while focusing simultaneously on the specific emotional issue through statements, clears energy blockages that might be obstructing our efforts to achieve our goals.

The following sequence, from Emma Roberts, takes just minutes and uses fifteen of the meridian points on the body; it is best to learn these off by heart (see diagram, p. 37). You'll need to learn:

❀ your 'set-up statement' (the phrase that you repeat)
❀ tapping the meridian points and the sequence
❀ the shortcut version.

Your set-up statement: This is not an affirmation because it does also acknowledge that there is a negative part to the process too – the part you are trying to shift. The statement runs as follows:

'Even though ------------, I deeply and completely love and accept myself.'

Both negative and positive ideas co-exist here. This allows for self-acceptance and stops unconscious self-sabotage. Our inner saboteur is a voice we are all familiar with – it's the one that says, 'Eat the chocolate cake!' when we are on a diet.

To do the set-up, take the first two fingers of one hand and tap on the side of your other hand where you would deliver a karate chop. You need to apply a little pressure – about as much as when someone gives you a prod. The aim is to send a vibration of energy down that point. As you tap on this point, say your 'set-up' statement out loud, including a specific issue you would like help with (anxiety, for example).

Repeat your statement three times. It may feel a bit odd the first time you try it. If you are really struggling with the 'I deeply love and accept myself' part, try 'I am OK' or 'I am good' to start with.

Tapping the meridian points and the sequence: You can tap with either hand, but it's probably easier to use your dominant one. Also, note the following:

- ✿ Tap using the tips of your index and middle fingers.
- ✿ Tap solidly, but never hard enough to hurt.
- ✿ Tap around seven times on each point.

The sequence is as follows:

- ✿ The eyebrow – at the beginning, just above and to one side of the nose.
- ✿ The side of the eye – on the bone, bordering the outside corner of the eye.
- ✿ Under the eye – on the bone, about 2.5cm below your pupil.
- ✿ Under the nose – on the small area between the bottom of your nose and the top corner of your upper lip.

❀ Chin – midway between the point of your chin and the bottom of your lower lip.

❀ Collarbone – at the junction where the breastbone, collarbone and first rib meet. To locate it, first place your forefinger on the U-shaped notch at the top of the breastbone. From the bottom of the U, move your finger down a centimetre towards your stomach, then to the left (or right) by a couple of centimetres. It is at the beginning of the collarbone.

❀ Under the arm – on the side of the body, at a point even with the nipple for men or in the middle of the bra strap for women.

❀ Below the nipple – for men, a couple of centimetres below the nipple; for women, where the bottom of the breast meets the chest wall.

❀ Top of the head – on the crown of your head, spanning both hemispheres.

❀ Thumb – on the outside edge, at a point even with the base of the thumbnail.

❀ Index finger, middle finger and little finger – on the side, at a point even with the base of the fingernail.

❀ Karate chop point.

Note: If you tap your sequence down the body, it makes it easier to remember.

MERIDIAN TAPPING POINTS

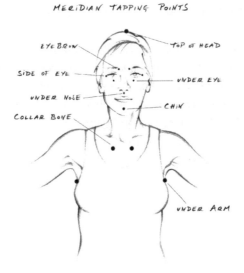

The shortcut version: This is as follows:

- ❀ Beginning of the eyebrow
- ❀ Side of the eye
- ❀ Under the eye
- ❀ Under the nose
- ❀ Chin
- ❀ Beginning of the collarbone
- ❀ Under the arm
- ❀ Top of the head

BALANCING YIN AND YANG

Yin is the cooling, moistening and calming aspect of our bodies, the part that lubricate 'the engine'. Yang is the activating and warming force in the body. We can see a connection with the nervous system in Western medicine in that it is also split into two parts – one concerned with regulation and one with action.

You may detect a deficiency of either Yin or Yang, and you can take gentle steps to rebalance these energies.

Yin Deficiency usually occurs in patients with severe Heat or in those who are seriously Blood Deficient. Yin Deficiency develops from overwork and/or failure to recover properly from a prolonged illness – it is a real burn-out condition.

Signs that Yin Deficiency has developed are Five Palm Heat, which is mild sweating in the palms of the hands, on the soles of the feet and a feeling of heat in the centre of the chest. Other symptoms include night sweats, feeling hot in the afternoon and a tongue that is either without coating or has shiny patches. The skin is often dry and shows early signs of ageing and the patient is often highly strung and anxious.

The following will help:

- No coffee
- No alcohol

- No smoking
- Lots of rest and relaxation
- Early nights
- Eating lots of Yin-nourishing foods, including apples, lemons, honey, eggs, tofu, seaweed, pork, pear, kidney beans and pineapple
- No skipping meals
- Meditation (see p. 64)
- Practising the ability to keep things simple and just 'be'
- Nurturing the ability to give love to yourself and practise acceptance

When Yang is deficient you lose your get-up-and-go and literally slow down. You may need to urinate more frequently and tend to find it very hard to lose weight. Even your thought processes will feel sluggish. Those with Kidney Yang Deficiency have a general lack of transforming energy which means there is a tendency to Coldness. The following will help, if this sounds like you:

- Lots of warming foods, including pumpkin, squash, reishi mushroom, cherry, black beans, tempeh, chestnuts, coconut, salmon, chicken, pheasant, turkey, milk, hawthorn, miso, molasses, ginger and brown sugar
- Moxibustion – this is warming (see p. 333)
- Movement and exercise
- Warmth and protection from the cold
- Allowing yourself to be passionate, inspired and engaged
- Practising 'doing'

Sleep Well

Getting a good, relaxed night's sleep is beneficial to your health, both in body and mind. Research has shown that insufficient sleep may harm your body's ability to heal and fight off illness.[5] It will affect your levels of focus and concentration, your moods and will feed into your stress levels.

In Chinese medicine, we interpret a lack of sleep as a factor which may deplete Qi, just like stress and overwork. And good sleep helps to build good Qi, essential throughout pregnancy.

What constitutes good sleep?

Western research suggests that between six and seven hours sleep is the minimum that will allow the body to experience the four essential stages of sleep, and that for adults between seven and nine hours a night is optimum.

I also place great emphasis on how you prepare for sleep – do you wind down in the hours before sleep or go to bed still buzzing from the day. You will know how long you need personally to feel well rested and energized on waking. Here are some suggestions to help you get a good night's sleep if you find it difficult:

Try to avoid:

- ❀ caffeinated drinks too late in the day – only drink coffee between 10 and 11 a.m., and in the evening stick with herbal teas like chamomile
- ❀ eating too late
- ❀ serious discussions close to bedtime
- ❀ working late
- ❀ sleeping pills – these may prevent the mind from experiencing all the four essential stages of sleep, which can leave you feeling more tired in the morning
- ❀ alcohol – this can have a similar effect to sleeping pills (see p. 53 for alcohol and pregnancy).

Do:

- ❀ go to bed early to avoid becoming overtired
- ❀ keep your bedroom as dark as possible
- ❀ give your brain a break before you go to bed; so spend some time taking a bath or doing relaxation exercises, rather than watching the TV or even reading
- ❀ keep electrical equipment to the bare minimum in your bedroom – these can produce electromagnetic energy which stimulates your brain while you're trying to sleep.

See p. 193 for more on sleep during pregnancy.

Exercise

As with work, I suggest a balanced approach to exercise as you prepare to make a baby and during pregnancy. Exercise is a wonderful way to get your Qi moving freely, and being in good shape when you conceive and during your pregnancy is beneficial to your health and your levels of energy and vitality. The key is to know your own level of fitness and moderate your exercise accordingly. Keep things gentle and stick well within your limits.

Yoga

If you haven't tried yoga before, this is a wonderful time to start. Yoga is the perfect exercise for any time of life, but especially before, during and after pregnancy. There is much focus on the breath, relaxation and flexibility, all extremely helpful. You can find yoga classes easily through your local gym or community centre, or there might even be a yoga centre in your area; see also Resources, p. 339.

Qigong

As suggested by the name, qigong (pronounced 'chee gong') is a Chinese form of exercise for building and improving the movement of Qi. It involves slow, graceful movements with controlled breathing techniques and is, therefore, both a form of exercise and meditation, beneficial to physical and emotional health. It is extremely good for releasing tension and stress as your body and mind become entirely focused on the movements and breathing. Check out your local paper or search online for classes in your area; see also Resources, p. 339.

Walking

This is the simplest, but one of the best forms of gentle exercise, especially if you are just starting to build up your fitness. Walking gets you moving in a forward direction, literally and metaphorically. If you are ever feeling a little stuck or low on energy, go for a walk; and the same goes for when you are feeling stressed or frustrated. Walking is the perfect distraction.

Your Environment

What we do to our environment we also do to ourselves. This is something I tell myself as a reminder that we are not separate from our environment, and that each of us has an individual responsibility to make the world a better place for the next generation.

So, given that this whole book is about improving health for the next generation, it's worth thinking about our immediate environment and how we can take steps to improve it. The challenge in this respect is that it is impossible to turn back time, and many of us wonder, therefore, if we can really make a difference. But while I have your attention, I'll say that it's worth making whatever difference you can; the links between your health and that of the environment are beginning to be more widely researched, and while we can't all live on an organic farm, we can take steps to reduce the chemicals in our own immediate environment.

Household cleaning products
I recommend choosing natural alternatives where possible – from brands like Ecover to using traditional natural cleaners like lemon and vinegar.

Insecticides and pesticides
These are dangerous to pregnant woman and should be avoided. You should also avoid them when trying to conceive.

Dry cleaning
Limit the amount of dry cleaning you have done to the minimum and take freshly cleaned clothes out of the plastic and air them before putting them away.

Cellophane and soft plastics
These can leak oestrogen-mimicking chemicals. Avoid plastic-bottled water where possible or transfer to another container. Be careful not to let plastic-bottled water heat up in the car.

Microwave
In Chinese medicine, the theory is that microwaves may affect the energy of natural foods, so are best to be avoided where possible.

Beauty products and treatments

Choose natural, organic products where possible. Avoid hair dyes, fake tans and most sun creams. Brands such as Dr Hauschka make chemical-free or reduced-chemical alternatives. Look for 'paraben-free' on the labels. And avoid Botox injections altogether.

Anti-perspirant

Use aluminium-free deodorants rather than anti-perspirants. Sweating is a natural process and a way for your body to eliminate toxins. Also avoid talc when you are trying to conceive as it can travel up the Fallopian tubes and affect the ovaries.

JING

One generation plants the trees, and another gets the shade.
Chinese proverb

Jing gives rise to life and is the blueprint you will hand down to your baby, through your genes and also through your pregnancy lifestyle and environmental factors in your life and theirs. As the sociobiologist Mary Jane West-Eberhard states from a Western perspective: 'Nothing is genetically determined in the sense of determined by genes alone. No gene is expressed except under particular circumstances.'[6] (So it's a case of nature *and* nurture, not one or the other.)

Prenatal Jing is what we inherit from our parents and postnatal Jing is what is cultivated through pregnancy, life and external factors. Postnatal Jing is the part we can influence.

Some people are born with incredibly strong Jing and can burn the candle at both ends, eat badly, drink like a fish and still hop out of bed in the morning with plenty of energy. Others need a more regular lifestyle to strengthen their Jing, and even the slightest deviation can upset the apple cart, leaving them feeling shattered. When God was giving out the genes it appears some did much better than others on the Jing front.

To gauge the state of the constitution you have inherited, answer the following:

- Was either of your parents older than thirty-five when you were conceived?
- Did either of your parents smoke at that time?
- Did they drink alcohol at around the time you were conceived?
- Did they take drugs?
- Did your mother smoke, drink or take drugs during pregnancy?
- Was your mother very stressed or traumatized during pregnancy?
- Was your mother ill during pregnancy?
- Did your mother have any serious accidents during pregnancy?
- Are you the youngest of many children conceived in quick succession?
- Did your parents suffer from any hereditary diseases?
- Do you have grey hair prematurely?

A poor inherited Jing can still be nourished and preserved by a moderate and well-balanced lifestyle, diet and attention to emotions. Foods such as seeds, congee (see p. 307), good-quality chicken stocks, algae and bee pollen are all said to nourish Jing.

Drugs, alcohol, chemicals, additives, pesticides and tobacco all deplete Jing, as do overwork and excessive sexual activity.

Smoking

Smoking has been shown to have a negative impact both on conception – smokers take longer to conceive – and on the ability to carry a pregnancy to term. Smoking during pregnancy may even impact on the reproductive systems of male foetuses.[7] The risk of damage to fertility is only slightly smaller for passive smoking than it is for active smoking. See Resources, p. 343, for help with quitting.

Recreational Drugs

All recreational drugs damage your chances of conceiving a baby, and also pose a serious threat to the development and health of your baby if you do conceive. See Resources, p. 343, for help.

*

Have you recognized any lifestyle or environmental factors you may want to tweak for fine-tuning your general health and well-being? Perhaps you would like to sleep more soundly, or you've realized that it's time to create more of a balance between work and other aspects of your life, especially as you are creating a family. Make a note of the things you would like to try. In the next chapter, we'll focus on diet and, even more importantly, digestion.

chapter three
IS THE FUEL GOOD?

Diet is important but digestion is everything.
Daverick Leggett

My definition of a healthy diet, based on the principles of Chinese medicine, is very simple. We can *eat for pleasure* in a way that also nurtures our health and vitality and not worry obsessively about how many calories or grams of fat or carbohydrate we are 'consuming'.

Food is a source of nourishment; it involves all our senses. Two people can eat the same meal and receive entirely different nourishment from it, depending on their digestion and state of mind. A healthy relationship with real food starts in the womb, before a child is even born. To eat well, eat light, live longer:

- ❀ Eat seasonal foods.
- ❀ Eat slowly and chew properly to aid digestion.
- ❀ Don't eat late at night.
- ❀ Eat organic food, where possible.
- ❀ In Chinese medicine, the stomach digests both thought and food – so try not to watch TV, study or read while you are eating, as this will take energy away from the efficient digestion of your food.
- ❀ Always eat a good breakfast.
- ❀ Drink when you feel thirsty – don't flood your system in the quest for eight glasses a day.

❀ Don't eliminate all fat – this is totally detrimental.

❀ Don't skip meals, as it will disrupt your blood sugars and play havoc with your hormones.

It's Not About Calories

In Chinese medicine, and indeed in Chinese culture, food is a healthy obsession. But rather than religiously working out a daily calorie intake, the obsession is with finding the freshest vegetables and creating dishes that provide the perfect balance for the body. It is a passion and a source of great pleasure. This simple desire to *eat well* is something that can have a hugely positive impact on our energy and sense of health and well-being.

Whether preparing for conception or during pregnancy, it is the perfect time to focus on eating well, both for you and your baby. It is then equally important to build this passion in the early days of motherhood and beyond. It's interesting that the biggest growth area in organic food is in baby food – giving our babies the best possible start in life that we can. Why not use this as a springboard to take care of your own health and nutrition too?

Developing a Healthy Relationship with Food

For many of my patients, their relationship with food is often more emotional than physical. They might eat for comfort, because a television advertisement suggests they will feel better if they eat a certain food, or to satisfy a craving. Many people have feelings of guilt around food and their ability (or otherwise) to say 'No'. Their sense of a healthy balance has gone out of the window.

I think it's a shame that food has become such a source of stress. Many women use food as a means of gaining control, when perhaps they might need to deal with emotional issues. It's helpful to remember that food is fuel for your body, and that if you listen to your body carefully, you'll instinctively make the right choices, especially during pregnancy. The core idea is to make subtle, sustainable shifts, rather than huge swings. If, for example, you decide you are a bit on the Hot side, you can gently start to introduce some Cooling foods (see p. 59). Small changes over time and made with ease are much better than radical, short-lived ones.

Balancing Our Food

A balance of carbohydrates, proteins and fats forms the foundations of our diet. In Western culture, it's incredibly easy for these foundations to fall out of a healthy balance because so much of our food is processed. In Chinese medicine, we consider the energy of food. There are some clear parallels with Western ideas of nutrition, so I will introduce the basics of Chinese medicine 'energetics' here and you'll see the similarities.

Grains

As in Western culture, grains form the foundation of the Chinese medicine diet and are the basis of Blood and Qi. They have a subtle sweetness that is nourishing, particularly to the Spleen, the engine of our digestion. They give us energy and 'scour' the intestines. Grains include: rice, oats, barley, rye, wheat, millet, amaranth, quinoa, buckwheat and corn.

Vegetables

Vegetables strengthen Qi, and eating a variety of leafy greens, root vegetables, watery vegetables and members of the onion family is excellent for general health and well-being. Root vegetables are naturally sweet and nourishing for the Spleen (great in the first trimester of pregnancy), while dark green leafies are rich in iron, and so are good for nourishing the Liver and Blood. Watery vegetables like cucumber are cooling for Heat conditions; think of the phrase 'cool as a cucumber'. And the onion family includes vegetables that are warming and pungent, helping to disperse Stagnation and prevent Dampness (this is mirrored in Western nutritional research suggesting the onion family is good for warding off colds).

Fruit

Fruit is supportive of Yin in that it is often moistening and cooling. It is not so good for Damp or Yang Deficiency, but often, warming fruit reduces the Dampening effects, which explains why warm compote on your porridge is so good during the autumn and winter months. Citrus fruits on the other hand are good for resolving Dampness.

Note: I encourage my patients not to eat fruit after a meal as it ferments in the stomach and slows digestion.

Beans and pulses

Beans are very nourishing and combine particularly well with grains and vegetables; in Western nutrition, beans and grains combine to create complete protein, especially useful for vegetarians.

Nuts and seeds

Nuts and seeds are concentrated in nourishment, so you need only a handful, but that handful is very good for Blood and Qi. Most nuts are Yin-nourishing, but there are also a few, including pistachio, chestnut and walnut, that are Yang-strengthening. They are excellent lightly toasted or roasted and scattered over dishes.

Dairy

In Chinese medicine nutrition, dairy foods are considered very rich, and consumed in excess they will have a tendency to create Phlegm or Damp. In Western nutrition, dairy foods are often associated with increased occurrences of asthma and sinusitis. However, in small quantities, these foods are deeply nourishing.

Meat and fish

Meat is the most Blood-nourishing of foods, acting as a tonic. Like dairy, it's good to have a little meat in your diet (unless, of course, you are vegetarian), but not too much, as it is then difficult for the digestion. Chicken is especially good for Qi, and I am somewhat obsessed by homemade chicken soup, recommending it to all my patients and anyone who will listen to me (see recipe, p. 314)!

Herbs and spices

The aromatic flavours of herbs and spices are stimulating to the Spleen and many, therefore, help with digestion. A lot of herbs and spices are warming, while some are cooling and they are used by cultures all over the world to bring balance to dishes. Herbs also make wonderful teas, from warming jasmine to cooling mint or soothing chamomile.

What's in our food?

It's an easy rule of thumb to follow that the more processed a food is, the more likely it is to contain little nutrition and to be of no major benefit to our overall health and well-being. Here's a short guide to the components of our food:

Fats

Fats are an important part of our diet, despite the negative associations often attached to them.

Monounsaturated fats

These have been shown to have a beneficial effect on cholesterol levels. They are found in:

❀ nuts, including walnuts, almonds, pistachios
❀ avocados
❀ olive oil.

Polyunsaturated fats

These include the two essential fatty acids (EFAs), omega-3 and omega-6. They are particularly beneficial to brain function (hence, fish really is brain food) and are anti-inflammatory. They can be found in:

❀ fish, including mackerel, salmon, trout and sardines (see p. 102) for how much fish to eat in pregnancy)
❀ sunflower seeds and oil
❀ flaxseed oil.

Saturated fats

Eaten in excess, these can raise cholesterol, and so it's best to eat in moderation. In Chinese medicine, we don't tend to think of these foods as 'good' or 'bad', and would instead describe these foods as rich – still good, but in small quantities. Saturated fats are found in:

❀ red meat
❀ egg yolks

- ❀ cheese
- ❀ coconut oil.

Trans fats

These are unsaturated fats (usually vegetable oils) that have gone through a chemical process which turns them from liquid into solid and causes them to act like saturated fats. Trans fats have been linked to high cholesterol and an increased risk of fertility problems.[8] I recommend avoiding trans fats wherever possible, which can be easier said than done, as there is no legislation currently which requires food manufacturers to declare trans fats in their ingredient lists. However, many supermarkets and producers are being open in their use of trans fats voluntarily, and you can also look for the term 'hydrogenated' fats in the ingredients as this is the process used to convert unsaturated fats into trans fats. These fats are often found in:

- ❀ chips
- ❀ fried foods
- ❀ biscuits and cakes
- ❀ margarines.

Carbohydrates

Carbohydrates provide us with energy and help with brain function. As with fats, not all carbohydrates are created equal when it comes to healthy nutrition.

Simple carbohydrates

Simple carbohydrates are those which act as sugars, including, of course, sugar itself and grains which have been refined to the point that they act just like sugar. Simple carbohydrates provide a quick burst of energy as they are broken down into glucose by the body very quickly. Unfortunately, that quick burst creates a spike in blood sugar, often followed by a low and a craving for another sugar fix. In Chinese medicine overconsumption of sweet foods leads to Dampness and damages the digestion. Simple carbohydrates include:

- ❀ sugar
- ❀ white rice

- ❀ white pasta
- ❀ white flour and bread
- ❀ packaged biscuits, chocolate bars and cakes
- ❀ fizzy drinks.

Complex carbohydrates

These are broken down more slowly by the body, providing sustained energy. They also supply another essential nutrient in our diet – fibre, which helps our digestive system to remove waste products, and acts as roughage to ease the way. In Chinese medicine, these foods form the foundations of all meals and include:

- ❀ whole grains, including brown rice, wild rice, quinoa, bulgur wheat, oats and spelt
- ❀ vegetables, including carrots, squash, pumpkin, swede, cauliflower and broad beans
- ❀ pulses, including lentils, chickpeas, adzuki beans and butter beans.

Water

Six glasses a day, eight glasses a day, two litres – the trend for making sure we drink vast amounts of water all day long is getting out of control. Water *is* essential, but – like anything else – you can have too much of a good thing, and disrupt your body's balance, including flooding your system with water from plastic bottles.

There is water in much of our food, especially fruit, vegetables, nuts and seeds. It's also good to get your fluid in a variety of ways, including herbal teas, soups and broths. In Chinese medicine, too much water stops the stomach from performing efficiently, diluting digestive enzymes and leaving food to sit in the bowel and ferment, which is never a good thing. So aim to strike a balance when it comes to fluid and your diet:

- ❀ Don't drink while eating.
- ❀ Avoid 'dry' foods – for example, eat fruit, nuts and seeds in the raw where possible, rather than toasted to a crisp.
- ❀ Soups are excellent (see p. 55) and good to include wherever possible.

❀ Don't drink water from the fridge, as the sudden contrast in temperature with that of your body will be hardening and constricting to your Qi. Drink warm or room-temperature water, and in the morning, add a slice of lemon for extra balancing qualities.

Herbal teas

The Chinese have enjoyed and revered tea for its medicinal properties for centuries. Happily, there is now a great deal of research that documents the various health benefits of tea. Most of the teas I suggest are caffeine-free or low in caffeine:

❀ Green tea (limit to 3–4 cups a day, due to caffeine content)
❀ Nettle tea
❀ Chrysanthemum flower tea (less well known, but can be found in most health-food shops)
❀ Dandelion
❀ Chai
❀ Ginger tea (soothing for some, but not if you have a tendency to Heat)

Coffee

There is much debate over whether coffee is good or bad for us. My view is that it is best avoided if you are preparing to make a baby, are pregnant or breastfeeding. It does stimulate the brain, digestion and the bowel and helps break down Stagnation (see p. 18) and Dampness (see p. 17). However, it is best avoided for those who are Blood Deficient, Yin Deficient or Heat. Too much caffeine has been linked to early miscarriage.[9]

Alcohol

In general, you should be thinking about absolute minimal alcohol intake. Although the current advice for pregnancy is to limit alcohol consumption to up to a small glass of wine a day, it is worth considering avoiding it altogether. Also, take note of the following:

❀ Never drink on an empty stomach. The liver can process alcohol more efficiently if you have eaten.

❀ Alcohol is a hormone disruptor, so if you suffer from thyroid problems, polycystic ovary syndrome (PCOS), endometriosis (see p. 68) or PMT, you should limit or avoid alcohol.

❀ Alcohol affects both male and female fertility, so is best avoided when trying to conceive.

Additives
There are a number of additives out there to be aware of and to avoid.

Monosodium glutamate (MSG)
This is an artificial food additive which has long been used in Asian food as a flavour enhancer and thickener. Studies show that MSG may contribute to fertility problems and affect the health of the unborn child. Look out for this ingredient on food labels and ask in restaurants if they use it.

Butylated hydroxyanisole (BHA)
This is less well known than MSG, but is used as a preservative in many foods, including butter, lard, meats, cereals, baked goods, sweets, beer, snack foods, processed meats and dry mixes for drinks and puddings. It is thought to mimic oestrogens and interfere with the menstrual cycle, so is best avoided if you are trying to conceive.

Aspartame
There is much debate over whether or not this artificial sweetener is bad for our health. It is usually added to anything 'diet' or 'sugar free'. Aspartame has been implicated in raising the risk of miscarriage. My advice is that it's not worth the risk, so avoid it.

Other additives to be avoided are:

❀ hydrolyzed protein
❀ hydrolyzed oat flour
❀ calcium caseinate
❀ sodium caseinate
❀ textured protein (including TVP)
❀ autolysed yeast.

The best way to avoid additives is to cook with fresh ingredients wherever possible and steer clear of processed foods. Keep it simple.

Weight-management Issues

According to guidelines from NICE (National Institute for Health and Clinical Excellence) published in 2010, 'Women should be encouraged to achieve a healthy weight before they become pregnant and advised that there is no need to "eat for two" when pregnant.'[10] The research suggests that not only are there greater health risks during pregnancy, but that babies of obese mothers will be more likely to become obese themselves later in life. It's important not to 'diet' while pregnant, but healthy eating and light exercise are important for all pregnant women; if you have struggled with weight, then as you become a mother it is the perfect time to look at making healthy changes to your lifestyle, both for your own benefit and your child's. Any positive changes will literally last a lifetime.

Just think of the challenge Jamie Oliver faced, trying to persuade schoolchildren to eat a healthier lunch. Even at five years old, habits and tastes are ingrained. Feed your unborn child with nutritious, healthy food during pregnancy, and you will strengthen their Jing, their constitution. They might even choose carrots over chips in the school canteen!

Seasonal Foods

In Chinese medicine, our bodies are connected with nature and its cycles. So the growing trend for eating seasonal foods isn't just a fashion, it really is good for you. Think about how warming soups and slow-roasted vegetables are so comforting during the autumn and winter months. Raw food during the spring and summer is also very helpful, balanced with lighter soups. Generally, in Northern Europe we need a diet that is warming and easy on the digestion, including whole grains, like barley and amaranth.

The Importance of Liquid Food

In China, no meal is complete without a bowl of soup, and I encourage all my patients to drink plenty of broths and simple soups. The Western diet has a tendency to be very dry from, say, muesli in the morning to sandwiches for lunch and many 'health' foods, like rice cakes and cereal bars. This has led to us trying to balance out the dry foods with gallons of water throughout the day. If you drink lots of water at lunchtime, all you are doing is flooding your digestive system, making it harder to digest the food.

The key is to find the right balance in the food itself, rather than compensate with bottled water. This is why soups and broths are essential, plus they are comforting and satisfying. They have a cleansing effect and while usually made of very simple ingredients are highly nutritious.

SQUASH

I encourage all my pregnancy patients to eat squash. It is so good for the digestion and Spleen and is a very versatile food: bake it, roast it, add it to soups, stews or risotto. Your Spleen will thank you for it!

Food Chart

In Chinese medicine, foods play very specific roles in terms of the Climates and nourishing the various organs, Qi and Blood. Often, the characteristics of certain foods come as no surprise; for example, that ginger is warming, cucumber is cooling and that meat nourishes the Blood. I refer to these food characteristics throughout the book, and so have included a simple chart you can use as an at-a-glance reference. If you are showing signs of Cold, I will encourage you to add warming foods to your diet; or if you are suffering from one of the common Damp conditions, it will be a good idea to avoid the Dampening foods.

Foods to nourish Qi

Almonds
Beef
Carrots
Cherries
Chickpeas
Coconut
Dates
Eggs
Figs
Grapes
Ham
Lentils
Mackerel
Milk
Millet
Molasses
Oats
Potatoes
Quinoa
Sage
Sardines
Sweet potatoes
Shiitake mushrooms
Squash
Trout
Venison

Foods to nourish the Blood

Adzuki beans
Apples
Apricots
Asparagus
Avocados
Beetroot
Black beans
Black sesame seeds
Blackcurrants
Cherries
Dates
Duck
Eggs
Honey
Kale
Nettle
Oats
Pears
Pomegranates
Pork
Royal jelly – fresh if
you can find it
Seaweed
Spinach
Sweet potatoes
Sweet rice
Tofu
Watercress

Yin-nourishing foods

Apples
Eggs
Honey
Kidney beans
Lemons
Pears
Pineapple
Pork
Seaweed
Tofu

Yang-nourishing foods

Anchovies
Basil
Cardamom
Cinnamon
Garlic
Lamb
Pistachios
Quinoa
Rosemary
Trout

Foods which resolve Damp

Adzuki beans
Asparagus
Barley
Basil
Buckwheat
Caraway
Cardamom
Celery
Coriander
Corn
Garlic
Green tea
Horseradish
Jasmine tea
Kidney beans
Lemons
Mackerel
Mushrooms
Onions
Oregano
Parsley
Pumpkin
Quail
Radishes
Rye
Turnips
Umeboshi plums

Foods which resolve Phlegm

Almonds
Apple peel
Black pepper
Celery
Garlic
Grapefruit
Lemon peel
Liquorice
Mushrooms
Olives
Onions
Pears
Peppers
Peppermint
Radishes
Seaweed
Shiitake mushrooms
Thyme
Watercress

Hot foods

Almonds
Beetroot
Brown lentils
Brussels sprouts
Cayenne pepper
Cinnamon
Cloves
Eel
Garlic
Ginger
Lamb
Peaches
Peppers

Warm foods

Blackberries
(cooked)
Carrots
Chicken
Chocolate
Cocoa
Coffee
Figs
Goat's milk
Greens
Mint tea
Oats
Onions
Oranges
Parsnips
Peanuts
Pumpkin
Radishes
Red beans
Sesame seeds
Indian tea
Tomatoes (cooked)
Turnips
Venison

Cold foods	Cool foods	Neutral foods
Apples	Aubergines	Broad beans
Bananas	Barley	Rice
Celery	Cow's milk	Coconut
Cottage cheese	Crab	Corn on the cob
Cucumber	Cress	Dates
Grapefruit	Green lentils	Eggs
Lettuce	Green tea	Grapes
Marrow	Lemons	Herring
Melon	Mung beans	Mushrooms
Mussels	Pork	Peas
Pears	Soft cheese	Potatoes
Yogurt	Soya milk	Plums
	Spinach	Runner beans
	Tofu	Strawberries
	Tomatoes (raw)	Veal
		Wheat
		White cabbage

Recipes

The recipes in this book are based on Chinese dietary principles, and so are designed to address different imbalances within the body. For example, someone who has too much Heat needs to eat Cooling foods, a nursing mother needs to eat foods that nourish the Blood and someone suffering from Stagnation needs ingredients which will move the Qi around the body. As well as trying the recipes I give you, I'd encourage you to play around with the ingredients in the lists above. So if you feel you are generally too Hot, for example, try to include as many Cooling foods as possible in your cooking. The important thing is not to get too bogged down in the detail though – you may identify strongly with a type, but you may not. So if you've simply had a day out in the cold and feel you need warming, use Warming ingredients; if you've spent the day on the beach, in the sun, try to have something Cooling to balance your energies. The more in tune you are with your needs, the less rigid you will be with this, as you will begin to trust your instincts.

chapter four
IS THE MIND ON BOARD?

To live long, people should take care not to worry too much,
not to get too angry, not to get too sad, not to get too frightened,
not to do too much, talk too much or laugh too much.
Sun Simiao

Your mind is such a powerful entity. If you can harness its power and make it work for you, almost anything is possible.

In Chinese medicine, the Heart is directly linked to the Womb, and each can impact on the other. It's vital to work through emotional issues wherever possible so that they don't hold you, or your health, back. It has always felt very natural to me that emotions should impact on health and that physical and emotional health are intimately connected. Chinese medicine has always resonated so deeply with me as this idea is at the very heart of it. Moreover, I have seen a growing acceptance of this idea across the whole field of medicine. I have been to many lectures and read countless books supporting the theory that the mind and the body are not separate, and the evidence is growing all the time.

Within my own practice, I see that although a patient may be described as not having a disease or illness, this does not automatically mean they are 'without suffering'. Much of the work I do is directed at 'calming the mind'; often, it is only when you get to the heart of what is emotionally wrong with a patient that you make any headway at all. There is a saying which I am often drawn back to: 'Unless you are treating the heart of the patient, you are not working deeply enough.'

The time now feels right for people to return to values that have become less fashionable in the past twenty years. Kindness, compassion, courage and patience are well in need of a revival. Pregnancy, and the journey it takes you on, is a perfect time to explore and reconnect to these values. I also think it is a good time to practise forgiveness and let go of deeply held grudges and resentments. Go on, have a go – you will feel the benefits for yourself and you will feel lighter for it.

Emotions and Health

Emotions are a part of being human. We all experience emotions of fear, upset, excitement, anger, grief and joy to a greater or lesser degree every day as we navigate through life. For women, emotions are often associated with our hormones, and so it's easy to begin to understand the close link between our emotional and physical health.

In Chinese medicine, when any one emotional state begins to dominate our behaviour and inner feelings, this disrupts our balance and the smooth flow of Qi. There are Five Emotions which, when in excess, trigger this imbalance – Anger, Joy, Worry, Sadness and Fear.

Anger affects the Liver

If you are easily upset or frustrated, and find it difficult to control your emotions, then anger is dominating. You might feel volatile or impulsive. (A great example of this is the frustration that builds up when you are stuck in a traffic jam.) Often, people work hard to control their anger, especially at work, and so appear composed on the surface but the stress is building underneath. They might feel like they are going to explode, and often do at the weekend, especially after a few drinks.

Joy is connected to the Heart

Joy is a wonderful emotion when in balance, and I encourage all my patients to let go of their fears and feel more joy, especially if they are experiencing problems with fertility. In excess, though, joy burns up all your energy reserves. This is when you start to seek pleasure and instant gratification constantly – you flit from one experience to the next without a moment's rest, needing more and more stimulation to feel the same amount of pleasure. It's like an addiction, and when the high wears off a person might feel anxious and alone, finding it difficult to sleep or relax. There's no middle ground – either you're up or you're down – and it's difficult to approach life with any sense of clarity.

The joy of a new baby is often mixed with anxiety over the responsibility involved, so we look to create a strong and grounded connection between the Heart and Womb throughout pregnancy.

Worry affects the Stomach and Spleen (digestion)

In this state, anxious, analytical thoughts take over and often stop you from taking action. Perfectionism replaces the freedom to enjoy creative thoughts and new experiences. In turn, boredom and apathy can set in, and a tendency towards lethargy and inertia. You can see how your energy might become stagnant in this state, leading to poor digestion, which affects the Spleen and Stomach, and a sense of heaviness in body and mind. You ruminate, over-think and overanalyse everything, often unable to action your thoughts. You can easily become self-absorbed, and so unable to absorb anything else.

Sadness affects the Lungs

If you start to let your life be ruled by a deep sadness, you will find you become overly defensive and keep anything personal at arm's length. You will likely be a control freak, maintaining everything in order and working away at acquiring success, while staying cool and detached. You might be judgemental when it comes to others who you see as a bit carefree and careless. You feel and act tight and buttoned up. It's important to let go and live a little; to learn from those who seem so free and easy.

Fear affects the Kidneys

When you live with the emotion of fear you find yourself always imagining the worst outcome, I know someone who calls this an 'impending sense of doom'. You live under a cloud, often very critical and cynical, and feel you can rely on no one but yourself. This is a hard-edged and cold emotion which prevents you from connecting with others, with life in general and with your own mind and body.

*

The first positive step is in recognizing if any of these emotions might be holding you back. You can then begin to work through any negatives and practise a few simple techniques that will bring your emotions back into a positive balance.

HOT-BLOODED

One particularly hot-blooded French patient of mine noticed a real change in her temperature after changing her heating activities and undertaking a course of acupuncture and herbs.

'Not only has my husband noticed that I am much calmer and less argumentative, but my best friend noticed a change in me too. Every year, for the whole of our lives, we have swum in the same waters. I am always the one to complain about it being so cold, and am the first to decline a swim in all but the hottest of weather. But this year, I ran straight in – the water felt completely different to me, but not to my friend, who said it was the same as it had always been.'

Normally, I would think it would be Cold people that dislike cold water, and that is certainly true; but this client was very Hot, so surely the water would be refreshing? I thought this over for a minute and then found a possible explanation. To a person with a great deal of Heat in their body, cold water can feel extremely cold, due to the contrast. But for a person with normal temperature (which she now was), the water is not such a shock as there is less of a contrast.

We are all made differently, but it does not mean we can never change with a small amount of fine-tuning.

Cultivation of the Mind

In Chinese medicine, working through the issues that hold you back is called cultivation of the mind. A similar concept in Western medicine is cognitive behavioural therapy (CBT). Peter Deadman, editor of the *Journal of Chinese Medicine*, cites that: There is ample evidence that avoiding intense negative emotions, calming the mind, laughing, generosity, all contribute to good health and longevity.[11]

Happiness and optimism have been shown to be beneficial to our health. It is also important to allow yourself to let go of negative emotions and tensions, release your anxiety. If you are someone who tends towards moaning, and find, once you start, that it's highly addictive, make a conscious effort to replace all that negativity with positive thoughts. Likewise, if you often compare yourself with others – rating your achievements against your peers or friends, never quite satisfied – then it's incredibly helpful to start to let go of this competitive streak. Pregnancies and indeed children are all individual, and comparisons only result in creating stress for all concerned.

Be thankful

This is an effective way to train your mind to focus on the positive: try spending five to ten minutes every day jotting down things you are grateful for, from the smallest detail, like a stranger giving up their seat on the train, to the big things, like love and good health.

Visualization

Visualization is a technique I use with patients throughout preparing to make a baby, pregnancy and during labour. I use it both to help women 'see' what is happening in their bodies and then imagine the outcome they desire – what the mind perceives the body conceives. I have included visualization exercises throughout the book, for pre-pregnancy, for each trimester and for preparing for birth and during labour. On their own or on conjunction with affirmations, these are a powerful way of connecting with your body.

Meditation on the breath

Meditation is used in many cultures for achieving inner calm. Our lives and our minds are often so busy they feel like a whirlwind. Thoughts shoot around at the speed of light, keeping us on high alert. The act of meditation can begin to slow these thoughts down, transform negative thoughts into positive and create a wonderful sense of relaxation. With practice, feelings of competition and anxiety are replaced by contentment and inner peace.

Inner silence is a tremendous calming technique you can use throughout the pregnancy process, and it's an effective way to maintain balance in your life in general. It's very settling; spending time with your thoughts allows you to recognize their patterns and those of your emotions, so that rather than ignoring or repressing them, you understand them.

As with visualization, you need to find somewhere quiet to practise. Just sit comfortably with your back straight and gently close your eyes. As thoughts drift into your mind, acknowledge them and let them drift away again. Breathe easily and evenly through your nostrils, focusing on how your breath enters and leaves your body. Concentrate on the breath and gradually, with practice, your mind becomes still and you feel calmer. I recommend doing this once a day for ten to fifteen minutes, increasing as you become more practised.

You can do meditation on its own or in conjunction with yoga. The ideal times of the day for practising are first thing in the morning and again in the evening. It's an incredibly effective way to get in touch with your thoughts and emotions.

When it comes to cultivation of the mind, the most important thing to remember is to find methods that appeal to you or to explore those that are a little bit out of your comfort zone. You may feel silly practising positive affirmations, for example, but it just might be the tonic you need; or you might be amazed at how good you feel thinking about doing nothing. I want to encourage you to invest time in valuing your thoughts and investigating your hopes, fears, ambitions and dreams, and then finding ways to deal with them or take action in ways you have never embraced before.

part two

PREPARING TO MAKE A BABY

Whether you are trying to conceive naturally or you are undergoing fertility treatment, the few months before you conceive give you an opportunity to fine-tune your diet and lifestyle to optimize your fertility and create the best possible environment for your baby's development during pregnancy.

In Chinese medicine, the links between the health of the parents and the health of their child are strong. You help to create the blueprint for your child's health through your own, and even if your lifestyle has been out of balance up to now, it will make an extremely positive difference if you prioritize your health at this time.

I also take a moment with my patients to remind them that fertility is a receptive act; it's not necessarily about achieving by *doing*. We're so used in our daily lives to striving for our goals, being the active participant at all times to attain our desire. While we can certainly do things to help create the right environment for conception, it's also a time to slow down, relax and simply *be*. Don't become so obsessed about timetables that you let the control freak in you take over. It's OK to keep things simple; in fact, it's a great Yin tonic.

The 28-day Plan

Your menstrual cycle can affect your mood, voice, behaviour, outlook on life and even whether men see you as attractive or not. Equally, it is affected by your health, diet, lifestyle, travel and changes in time zone.

In this section, I hope to put you back in touch with your natural, healthy cycle; if I can help you balance your body and mind throughout it, then you have a good chance of conceiving. Women often arrive at my clinic with negative associations related to their periods. The arrival of a period may signal spots, bloating, sore breasts, high emotions and cravings for sugary comfort foods, like chocolate and cake. You may have to endure cramps, dose up on painkillers and moan to anyone who will listen.

I want you to begin now to let go of the negative associations with your menstrual cycle. Your hormones play an important part in your health – your periods are a real guide to how you are feeling generally and, of course, they are intrinsically linked with your fertility: your period signals a new beginning each month, releasing hormones that stimulate your maturing eggs, one of which will be released during ovulation around fourteen days later.

Hormones are at the heart of your cycle, creating natural periods of energy, creativity and quieter times for nurturing and relaxing. Once you understand the way you feel at different times, you can begin to understand just what is happening in your body during the cycle. And if your life is generally balanced and healthy, you will find it much easier to cope with nature's ups and downs. You will see the difference in your mood, energy and menstrual bleed (since this is the outward manifestation of the changes taking place in you).

It's helpful to keep a diary of your menstrual cycle at this time, so that you will be able to make small adjustments to fine-tune your health in preparation for conception. In an ideal world, I'd recommend a four-month pre-conception plan. Four months is the time it takes for the eggs to become mature in the ovaries. From experience with my patients, if you can help out your body during this time, then the likelihood of a positive outcome increases and can also have an equally positive effect on your general sense of well-being. A plan of action is also very helpful during this process – it helps to manage stress and moves you away from the stop-start of focusing purely on the time between your period and ovulation. This is a time to think about your health and fertility as a whole, rather than for a few days every month.

As I go through the stages of your cycle, I encourage you to visualize what is happening at each stage (I will do this throughout your pregnancy too). You will see your eggs ripening, your endometrium (womb lining) thickening, the egg releasing from the follicle and then implanting. As you read these descriptions, imagine your body effortlessly completing each stage.

CASE STUDY

EASING THE PAIN

Greta had such severe endometriosis that she had to take two days off work every month around her period. After two months of changing her diet and receiving acupuncture, she reduced her painkillers and only needed one day off. After four months, she had one day of mild pain, needed no painkillers and no longer took any days off work. This was after ten years of suffering.

chapter five
DAYS 1–5: DURING YOUR PERIOD

Begin a menstruation diary the day you start your period. Mark it in your diary as Day 1. If you start in the late afternoon or evening, the following day is considered Day 1.

Is the Engine Working?

Ideally, menstruation begins with a light flow of red blood, followed by the main flow, which is a little heavier, within twenty-four hours. Your period should be without clots, without pain and it should last an average of four to five days. There should be no spotting after your cycle. If this doesn't quite fit your description of your own period though, don't worry. If you follow my basic advice and the specific, symptom-related advice below, you should start to fall in with the 'ideal' cycle within a couple of months.

The diary is an essential tool as it will help you to chart how you feel and whether changes are happening. Many of my patients look and feel significantly different within just a couple of months and feel empowered, rather than slaves to their hormones.

RECOMMENDATIONS FOR ALL
Do:
- take things easy and go to bed early as often as possible
- use bergamot, chamomile and cypress oils, as they are excellent for menstrual pain – pour a few drops into your bath or dilute with a carrier oil (such as almond) for massage
- take Epsom-salt baths (see box below)
- as far as possible, keep your emotions calm and relaxed and don't get embroiled in any rows
- invest time in ideas, plans and being creative – this is a time of renewal and clarity of vision
- practise yoga or qigong.

Don't:
- use tampons at all, ideally, as they can cause Stagnation of Blood (because they don't absorb the clots which then travel back inside the uterus); I realize this can be difficult though, so try to limit your use and don't use them at night (you might want to use the Mooncup – a reusable menstrual cup made from soft medical-grade silicone; see Resources, p. 343)
- have sex – this, again, can cause Stagnation of Blood
- swim during your period as Cold can easily penetrate.

EPSOM-SALT BATH
Adding Epsom salts to your bath is a great way to relieve many menstrual discomforts:
- Pour four cups of Epsom salts into your bath water.
- Soak for twenty minutes.
- Try to lie down and rest for fifteen minutes following your bath.

PROBLEMS WITH MENSTRUATION

There are many medical reasons that may be the cause of problems with periods. From a Chinese medicine perspective, we look to address potential imbalances. Read through Part One to ascertain which tendencies you have and how to adapt your diet and lifestyle to help get things back into balance. **Note:** Always go and see your doctor if your periods stop.

Amenorrhoea (no periods) This can be caused by Blood Deficiency, Blood Stagnation or Damp.

Metrorrhagia (heavy or prolonged periods) This can be caused by Heat or Blood Stagnation, and also (although less so) by Qi Deficiency.

Dysmenorrhoea (painful periods) This can be caused by any of the conditions: Cold, Damp/Heat, Blood Deficiency and Blood Stagnation.

Is the Fuel Good?

Don't comfort-eat or eat to suppress emotions. Keep meals simple and, if you suffer from bloating and digestive disturbances, consider food-combining, so that you keep proteins and carbohydrates separate. For example, if you eat meat, have it with vegetables and, likewise, if you have grains, eat them with vegetables, rather than with meat. Add citrus peel to vegetable or meat dishes and include plenty of the following in your diet:

- ✿ Squash and other root vegetables
- ✿ Onions
- ✿ Fennel
- ✿ Watercress
- ✿ Coriander
- ✿ Dill
- ✿ Pickles with a meal
- ✿ Chamomile tea
- ✿ Jasmine tea

Thyme tea

Thyme is a herb with many healing properties and, specifically, it may help with relieving period pain and treating infections like thrush. Simply make a pot of tea with a handful of fresh thyme, steep for five to seven minutes and drink either hot or cold.

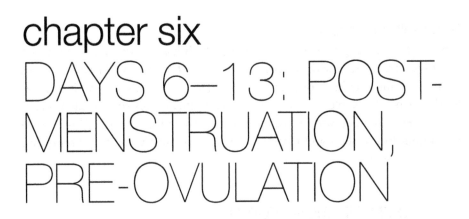

chapter six
DAYS 6–13: POST-MENSTRUATION, PRE-OVULATION

This crucial part of the cycle is called the follicular phase. It is also the week when you often feel most naturally creative, productive and positive. Both physically and mentally, this is a time of growth.

Is the Engine Working?

Anything around twenty-seven and thirty-one days is a normal cycle, although if you experience a very regular thirty-two or twenty-six day cycle, for example, that may well be 'normal' for you. Travel, emotional stress and illness can all alter the length of the menstrual cycle, so factor in any major disruptions and take an average. If you are experiencing either a long or short cycle then it's worth focusing some extra effort on this week of your cycle. If you are unable to lengthen or shorten your cycle with my advice, you will need to work with your GP or specialist.

Long follicular phase

This is when the egg is released too late in the follicular phase. In some women, it takes longer for the follicle to mature and the knock-on effect is that the whole cycle is slightly longer. Sometimes, the egg is mature, but does not release on time due to Stagnation. This is usually caused by anxiety or tension, so try to relax and enjoy yourself at this stage of your cycle. Make the most of your energy and creativity.

Short follicular phase

This is when the egg is released too early, which has the knock-on effect of a short menstrual cycle, with the period coming between Days 21 and 24. This is often because the hormones are out of balance – the egg may well be ferti-lized, but not be viable. In Chinese medicine, this relates to too much Heat, usually generated because the Yin is deficient. Introduce plenty of Yin- (cool) nourishing foods (see Food Chart, p. 56) and follow my advice for removing Heat (see p. 31).

RECOMMENDATIONS FOR ALL
Do:
- eat foods to nourish the Blood (see Food Chart, p. 56)
- practise meditation for keeping calm (see p. 64)
- be a free spirit and express yourself creatively – this is an excellent time for new projects
- if you are feeling productive, go ahead, but don't wear yourself out
- drink nettle and raspberry-leaf teas
- use rose and geranium essential oils at this time
- make hay and make sex a priority at this time.

Avoid (where possible):
- alcohol
- tobacco
- caffeine
- air conditioning
- too much heating
- too much computer time
- spicy foods
- medication for hay fever (can dry fertile mucus).

Is the Mind on Board?

The follicular phase is an especially powerful time to start new and creative projects.

Visualization

Your reproductive system is continuing its well-synchronized dance. The follicles are swelling, producing increasing amounts of oestrogen, while the ripening egg is preparing to burst into the Fallopian tubes. In the womb, the first layers of the endometrium are being laid.

RECOMMENDATIONS FOR MEN

Do:

- take charge of your sexual health – make sure you see your doctor if you suspect you may have any STDs or low-grade infections
- lose any excess weight
- take regular exercise
- take zinc supplements
- talk to your doctor if you take the antidepressant Paroxetine (also known as Seroxat or Paxil) – research suggests that it increases the levels of sperm with damaged DNA
- cut down on alcohol
- avoid heat (steam rooms, for example)
- avoid unfiltered city tap water
- avoid toxic paints, paint stripper and paint-diluting chemicals.

Don't:

- smoke cigarettes or marijuana
- take recreational drugs
- use your laptop on your lap
- keep your mobile phone in your trouser pocket, next to your testicles
- try to conceive shortly after an anaesthetic.

chapter seven
DAY 14:
OVULATION

The miracle of the moment of conception is just that – a miracle. Western medicine struggles to explain *exactly* how the meeting of sperm and egg can create the brand new cell of a separate being.

On Days 12 and 13 of a twenty-eight-day cycle, FSH (follicle-stimulating hormone) and oestrogen levels rise high enough for the process of ovulation to begin. The pituitary gland releases more LH (luteinizing hormone) which stimulates one (occasionally more) ripened egg to rise to the surface of the follicle.

On Day 14, the egg bursts through the protective follicle, propelled by the release of prostaglandins, and is released into the adjacent Fallopian tube.

Around ovulation, we all get a little flirty – it's official. Research has shown that our faces, scent and voice all become more attractive when we reach our fertile period, and our bodies increase production of oestrogen to facilitate ovulation. We even become more confident, have more energy, a heightened sense of smell and are definitely more interested in having sex, helpfully.

When everything is in good working order, you have a 30 per cent chance of conceiving during ovulation. To work out when you are ovulating, look for increased vaginal secretions: this cervical or 'fertile' mucus is produced to help the passage of the sperm. Healthy, clear cervical mucus, like egg whites, is a sign you are about to ovulate and that you are fertile. If your mucus is thick and yellow, this could indicate Damp/Heat; if it is thick and white, this could indicate Damp/Cold (see p. 31); and if it is scanty or absent this can indicate Blood Deficient or Heat (see p. 33).

RECOMMENDATIONS FOR ALL
Do:
- concentrate on building Qi (see p. 26)
- use meditation to avoid getting stressed (see p. 64)
- use the essential oils lavender, rose, ylang ylang, neroli and melissa – they all help the Heart–Womb connection which brings about a feeling of harmony and wholeness (see p. 90)
- drink chamomile tea – it is calming and will help you stay balanced
- try pelvic drainage abdominal massage (see box below) to invigorate Qi and blood in the abdomen
- increase your intake of essential fatty acids (see p. 50)
- start increasing sex on about Day 10 and for a few days after ovulation.

Don't:
- drink too much water
- use lubricants.

PELVIC DRAINAGE ABDOMINAL MASSAGE
Use massage oil (such as olive or almond oil mixed with a few drops of tangerine or bergamot oil). Massage along the bikini line and then, with a light technique, sweep the fingers from the pubic bone to the tip bone on the left side and then the right. This is decongesting for the pelvic region and can help with movement and release of an egg.

Not Ovulating?

If you are not ovulating regularly (often this is the case in women with polycystic ovary syndrome – PCOS), I would use acupuncture points on the abdomen and over the ovaries, attached to an electro-acupuncture machine, which is also attached to points on the ankle that relate to the reproductive system.

It is also helpful to practise visualizing the egg releasing at the same time as developing the Heart–Womb connection (see p. 90).

OVULATION TEST STICKS

Ovulation sticks measure the levels of luteinizing hormone (LH) in the urine. When there is a 'surge' this indicates the egg is about to be released.

Ovulation sticks can be helpful if you:

- have an irregular cycle and aren't sure when you are ovulating
- don't notice any changes in cervical mucus at this time
- are wondering if you are ovulating at all.

However, they are not helpful if:

- you are worried about ovulation – they can cause unnecessary additional stress
- you rely on them rather than listening to your own body
- they put too much focus on the time of ovulation, rather than sex and intimacy around the entire cycle; they can also add pressure and tension to sex.

Signs of not ovulating are

- ❀ no periods
- ❀ very irregular periods
- ❀ blood test shows low oestrogen/progesterone levels or high FSH.

Is the Mind on Board?

Visualize your ovary releasing the egg easily and freely. Imagine your body letting go, breathe freely and deeply and relax.

chapter eight
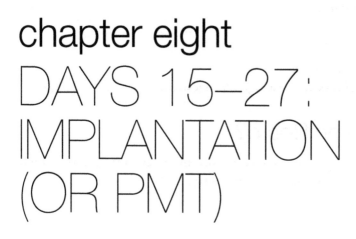
DAYS 15–27: IMPLANTATION (OR PMT)

If you are trying to conceive, these two weeks can seem like the longest imaginable. I want you to practise mental strength, patience, meditation and yoga during this phase to distract you from your preoccupation with conception, which can otherwise become all-consuming.

What Is Happening?

For implantation to take place, three things need to occur: a good-quality egg has to be released, fertilization between the egg and sperm must take place to produce an embryo and the womb lining has to be the correct thickness.

Days 15–22

The follicle that released the egg continues to produce oestrogen and progesterone, preventing any of the other follicles from producing eggs. These hormones are crucial to very early pregnancy and will help maintain the egg if fertilized. In the uterus, the endometrial lining is thickening and begins to produce nutrients in preparation for implantation.

Days 22–24

This is when implantation of the embryo may take place. You may also experience a little blood spotting after implantation, which is sometimes confused with the onset of menstruation.

Days 25–27

If the egg is not fertilized and, therefore, implantation does not take place, the corpus luteum (what is left of the follicle after ovulation) disintegrates and is absorbed. Oestrogen and progesterone levels then drop, causing the build-up of the uterus lining to fall away as the menstrual flow. The unfertilized egg will be passed out in your menstrual bleed.

Simultaneously, the pituitary gland starts to produce the hormones needed to stimulate the ripening of the next cycle's eggs in the ovaries.

PMT

PMT (premenstrual tension) is an umbrella term for a range of symptoms, the most common of which are cramps, backache, headache, the urge to cry, tiredness, depression and irritability. These discomforts are caused, in part, by prostaglandin hormones, essential for the menstrual cycle and also for labour. They travel through the bloodstream and can, unfortunately, cause pain elsewhere in the body.

Natural remedies

- One of the most effective supplements for PMT has been shown to be evening primrose oil. It helps to balance the hormones and therefore treats the cause rather than the symptom.
- Other studies have shown the benefits of eating foods with a low glycaemic index (GI). These foods release energy into your bloodstream at a slow pace rather than causing spikes to your blood-sugar levels. Examples are oats, whole grains, leafy green vegetables, beans and pulses.
- Address issues of the mind. Where the Qi is Stagnant, there is always emotional involvement.

Carrot, Ginger and Cashew Sweet Mood Muffins

This is an excellent premenstrual recipe, good enough to lift even the moodiest of days. If we all ate these on a few days of the month the world would be a much more pleasant place. The spices are gently warming and moving, exactly what the body needs to keep things flowing and counteract the dampening effects of the sugar and wheat. The oats and carrots are good hormone regulators and, along with the spices, ease any digestive or reproductive spasms that can lead to pain with a large dose of comfort!

Makes 12

275g (9¼oz) carrots (about 5 medium)
75g (2½oz) oat bran
65g (2¼oz) plain flour
60g (2oz) wholemeal flour
150g (5½oz) sugar or 120ml (4fl oz) agave syrup (a little more for decorating)
1 teaspoon caraway seeds, lightly crushed
1 teaspoon dried ginger
1 teaspoon cinnamon
¼ teaspoon cardamom
2 teaspoons baking powder
¾ teaspoon bicarbonate of soda
½ teaspoon salt
115–170g (4–6oz) plain yogurt
60g (2oz) unsalted butter, melted
1 large egg
115g (4oz) raw cashew nuts, chopped
orange zest or orange marmalade for decoration

1. Preheat the oven to 190°C/375°F/gas mark 5. Line 12 cups of a standard muffin tin with paper liners.
2. Wash and peel the carrots. Using a food processor or by hand, grate the carrots and place them in a colander or sieve over a bowl to drain any liquid. Set aside.

3. In a big bowl, mix together the oat bran, flours, sugar or agave, spices, baking powder, bicarbonate of soda and salt, and set aside.
4. In another large bowl, whisk together the yogurt, butter and egg. (If you have used agave, you may only need 100g/3½oz yogurt; you're looking for a sticky, slightly spongy texture – use an ice-cream scoop to test.)
5. Make a well in the centre of the dry ingredients, and add the yogurt mixture. Lightly stir until just combined, then stir in the cashews and fold in the carrots (leaving out any excess liquid). Spoon the mixture into the prepared muffin tin (or a loaf tin, if preferred).
6. Top each muffin with a few pieces of orange zest and a drop of agave or a dusting of sugar or a small dollop of marmalade. (Spread over the top of the loaf.)
7. Bake for about 45 minutes until firm and springy to touch. Transfer to a cooling rack and serve warm or at room temperature.

Is the Engine Working?

This is the Yang phase of the cycle, traditionally a time for 'warming the Womb'. During the Yang phase, I treat those who are trying to conceive differently from those who are not. When trying to conceive, the treatment needs to be very gentle. I always assume conception has taken place, and my aim is to support the pregnancy, rather than try to rectify any tendencies. So, if someone has Cold tendencies I would still be warming them, but gently.

RECOMMENDATIONS FOR ALL

Yang is warming in essence so you can support this warming process yourself. Western medicine often treats this phase of the cycle using progesterone, which also has a warming function. Women with tendencies of Heat or Yin Deficiency won't need so much warming though as they already have enough Heat or Yang for this phase.

Do:

- eat warming foods, such as ginger, little and often – the key is not to let your blood sugar drop
- rest well during this phase
- wear socks in bed if it's very cold outside
- keep your lower back warm – I recommend a 'kidney warmer' where you simply tie a cotton scarf loosely around your waist with particular attention to the lower back
- moxa on Stomach 36 (St 36) (see p. 112)
- practise positive visualization of what is going on in the uterus.

Don't

- sit in draughts
- take vigorous exercise
- overwork or get stressed
- walk barefoot on cold floors
- get too cold if you go swimming
- use microwaves.

Is the Fuel Good?

Limit your fruit intake (unless cooked with warming spices like apples with cinnamon). The exception is fresh pineapple, which is high in the enzyme bromelain; this may aid implantation due to its ability to thin the blood.

- ❀ Slow-cook your food – baking and roasting are good.
- ❀ Drink chai, cinnamon, ginger and cardamom teas.
- ❀ Balance raw foods with something warm.
- ❀ Avoid cold drinks, and drink water at room temperature rather than chilled.
- ❀ Avoid stodgy carbohydrates.
- ❀ Avoid fats – except for monounsaturated fats and EFAs (see p. 50).

Is the Mind on Board?

As you go through your cycle, I urge you to think about your own needs and get in touch with your creative side – whatever brings you joy. Sometimes these 'fertile' activities nourish us on an emotional level and literally make us more fertile. This post-ovulation phase is a particularly powerful time to start new creative projects.

In the Yang phase I also concentrate on mental strength, with particular emphasis on banishing fear:

❀ Don't give in to fear or doubt, and practise forgiveness.
❀ Transform fears into positives.
❀ Find your inner strength, resilience and your 'spark'.
❀ Use this as a time for quiet reflection and evaluation.

Throughout your journey, try to keep in mind the importance of preparation and the gift of good health you will be passing on to your baby. It may take a little time to conceive your longed-for dream, but all the while, you are gaining health and learning patience, both of which are good foundations for creating fertile soil.

part three
PREGNANCY

This is the one of the most exciting and terrifying changes you and your body will ever go through. There is so much going on inside your bump, and your thought processes are probably all over the place.

The first thing to say is, whatever you are feeling, the chances are it is normal. Remember, pregnancy is how all of us got here, but no matter how many have gone before you, you are pretty special and it is still incredible. So take your time and don't expect too much of yourself. You will feel mixed emotions and there is nothing wrong with that; allow yourself to adjust gradually to the miracle that is pregnancy.

I am not here to replace your healthcare professional – I believe that pregnancy is the domain of the midwife or, in some cases, the obstetrician. I am here to support you, and as an adjunct to these professionals' care of you.

In the course of the following chapters, I am going to take you through the various stages of pregnancy, known as trimesters. At the beginning of each chapter, I will ask you to focus on the development of your baby and what's happening to your own body. I want you to do this not only because it is interesting, indeed, miraculous, but also because by knowing what is happening to your body and to your baby, you can be more aware. You can use it as a meditation: read the passage referring to where you are in your pregnancy, then lie down quietly and picture the image of your baby growing inside you. Don't worry if you don't feel you want to do this though; you will find your own way to connect and bond with your baby. And really, that is the point of all of this: to find your own way.

But one of the reasons why I want you to be more aware is so that you can prevent minor pregnancy conditions from becoming more serious. Be your own health detective and listen to your instincts as you keep this book close at hand. I have simplified the ideas of Chinese medicine in order to make them accessible, remaining true to the essence, I hope, without going into too much technical detail. If you find that you fall in love with Chinese medicine, there are several books in the Further Reading section that I have recommended (see p. 347).

Of course, many people sail through pregnancy with not so much as swollen ankles. Others are not quite so lucky though, and seem to suffer and never quite get to the blooming stage. It is important not to compare yourself to others, we are all born different and when they handed out the genes (or for the purposes of this book, the Jing), some definitely did better than others. I have set this section out so that however you are feeling, you will be able to get something from it. So if you want to work through it and try to stay in shape so that you avoid conditions from developing, you can do that; or, if you are already suffering, you can go straight to the relevant page for some quick tips to help you out.

Lastly, be positive; don't let other people's thoughts or judgements affect you too much. They may mean well, but sometimes just manage to say the wrong thing.

CHINESE MEDICINE AND PREGNANCY

The first important point to make is that pregnancy is not said to cause any problems to a woman's health. In fact, there are certain conditions that actually improve during pregnancy. Many women who suffer from migraines say they loved pregnancy as they were migraine-free for nine months. However, some conditions, and by that I mean things like Blood and Yin Deficiencies, can be made worse. So not only is it important to prepare for pregnancy so that you start from a good place of health, it is also important to take care during pregnancy.

The type of energy imbalances that I often see during pregnancy from a Chinese medicine viewpoint are:

- Blood Deficiency – which can progress to Yin Deficiency
- Qi Stagnation
- digestive (Spleen) weakness – leading to Phlegm.

The principles of treatment are to:

- nourish the Blood (and Yin)
- move Stagnation of Qi
- strengthen the digestion (Spleen) and eliminate Phlegm.

Many of the pregnancy conditions I see in clinic are caused by one or a combination of the above disharmonies. Much of the advice in the following chapters is directed at preventing them from occurring in the first place.

At this point, I think it is worth reintroducing some of the organs that are commonly involved. You will remember that when I talk about the organs in Chinese medicine they are written with a capital letter (the organs have a wider influence and meaning here than in Western medicine). The Liver, for example, is connected to the eyes and the tendons, and is associated with the emotion of anger and frustration. So when I mention the Liver, you know I mean more than just the large organ under your right rib cage. It does not mean there is anything physically wrong with your liver from a Western medicine perspective, but it does mean you may begin to see the links between the emotional and physical associations with the Liver.

Liver

The Liver helps move the Qi and Blood around the body, which is very important to the correct development of your baby. Your pregnant body requires a good flow of blood to the uterus which nourishes and sustains the baby. The Liver is responsible for circulation and so benefits from movement. As I mentioned above, Qi Stagnation is something that pregnant women commonly suffer from and it can occur as pain, indigestion with bloating and gas. It may also be caused by unresolved issues and show in the mood as irritability and frustration. A sign that the Qi is Stagnant is sighing, which reflects Qi that is stuck in the chest, often from repressing emotions or not saying what we want to say. You need to learn to express yourself appropriately for the sake of your Liver.

Kidneys

It is said that the Kidneys store our Jing (see p. 16), which is important both to our own health and that of our children. Good, strong Kidneys are a sign of good health and a strong constitution. If the Kidney energy is weak, you may experience problems with the lower back, with urination, oedema (see p. 211) and you may feel emotionally very fearful (see p. 146). The Kidney energy is said to decline with age. In my experience, however, I see many pregnant women in their late thirties who take care of themselves and their well-being and have good Kidney energy.

Heart

The Heart and Womb are connected via an internal channel and so we can see the strong link between a woman's emotions and her fertility. This explains why your emotions could affect the baby growing inside you.

In clinic, I see many women who have tried for a long time to conceive, and when they are at last pregnant, many are scared to hope in case it goes wrong. However, I always say, 'Put your Heart into it and allow yourself to have hope.' If you don't put your Heart into pregnancy, you sever the connection between the Heart and the Womb when you need it the most (see Heart and Womb exercise, p. 97). Instinct, compassion and the ability to feel joy are all important Heart attributes.

Spleen and Stomach

These are the all-important organs of digestion. For too long now we Westerners have been totally fixated on diet – but, generally speaking, we don't pay enough attention to the digestion. As the Chinese medicine mantra goes: 'Diet is important, but digestion is everything.'

For good digestion, you need to look after the Spleen and the Stomach. This means not flooding the digestion with gallons of water and not living like a rabbit on a diet heavy in raw food. This view often makes me unpopular, but I see women who follow this diet to the extreme in the belief that they are being healthy, but in reality, their digestive function is often poor and their systems too Cold. I also see people who overindulge, then go on extreme diets in the hope that they will lose weight or 'get healthy'. In reality, balance and moderation provide a far healthier approach.

When the digestive fire is weak, then Dampness and Phlegm are generated, with all the associated problems we see with them. Worry and anxiety are the emotions of the Spleen and Stomach, and if you ruminate about everything and habitually overthink, this denotes a weakened digestive function. Being obsessed about self and also about diet suggest an imbalance of the Spleen.

I often see in my own practice how the majority of so-called 'minor' pregnancy ailments can be addressed with acupuncture and subtle lifestyle adjustments. And, by understanding how a person might become ill, we are given a window of opportunity where we are often able to prevent a condition from starting or from becoming more entrenched and, therefore, more difficult to treat.

Lack of energy, aches and pains, general malaise and acid heartburn are all conditions for which Western medicine has little to offer, but to the acupuncturist are at the very essence of what we do every day. Most acupuncturists will regularly treat women with morning sickness. We frequently turn breech babies into the head-down position for women who would otherwise have C-sections. We make people feel more energetic, less stressed and worried, and we give them a safe way to manage their health issues.

chapter nine
FIRST TRIMESTER (WEEKS 1–12)

A normal pregnancy will last between thirty-seven and forty-two weeks, an average of forty weeks from the first day of your last period. As I said, dividing a pregnancy into thirds, trimesters, is a helpful way to follow your own and your baby's development. The first trimester is from weeks 1 to 12, the second trimester from weeks 13 to 27 and the third from weeks 28 to 40.

Is the Engine Working?

From the moment of fertilization to week 12, your baby will develop at amazing speed, considering how complex the human body is.

How your baby develops

Your pregnancy actually begins in week 3, as pregnancies are dated back to the first day of your last period, while conception takes place around two weeks later. When the sperm penetrates the outer surface of the egg, fertilization occurs and cell division begins, one into two, into four, into eight . . . As this process begins, the egg is moved by the cilia (tiny hairs) along the Fallopian tube towards the uterus.

By the end of week 3 – so about a week after fertilization – the egg is now a tiny ball of around a hundred cells, just visible to the naked eye at 0.15mm diameter and described as a blastocyst.

After four weeks, the blastocyst has implanted itself in your uterine wall and begins to make its presence known to your body. In turn, your body responds by producing hormones that create the perfect environment for pregnancy. The inner cells develop into the embryo and the outer cells into the placenta. The foundations of development are being laid even now, as the cells begin to form into three groups, which will eventually become the skeleton, nerves and vital organs.

Over the next week, the embryo develops tiny ridges along the 'back' that will form the spine. The head is just beginning to develop, as are the brain and spinal cord. Right now, the embryo resembles a tiny sea horse.

From six weeks begins a period of crucial development. Slight depressions on the head show where the eyes and ears will be, the lower jaw is starting to become distinct and the arms and legs are just beginning to grow, although just tiny bumps at this stage. The inner layer of cells start to specialize into the internal organs, including the lungs, liver, stomach, intestines and bladder, and the blueprint for the baby's nervous system has been formed.

At Week 7, the embryo is approximately 1.5cm. The beginnings of the eyes are just visible beneath the surface and the ends of the arms are rounded and have impressions where the fingers will be. Inside, the heart has formed two chambers and the brain has also divided into the two hemispheres.

By Week 8, the embryo is about the size of a peanut and is now known as a foetus. Elbow and knee joints have appeared and the fingers are becoming more defined. The foetus can make tiny movements now, but you wouldn't feel them yet.

By Week 10, all the body parts are present, if not fully developed. The placenta will be fully formed and transport nutrients from you to your baby.

By Week 11, the critical period of *development* which has occurred over the past few weeks ends and a phase of dramatic *growth* begins, including the limbs, spine, ribs and genitalia. The heart is so well developed that it now pumps the baby's own blood around the body.

By twelve weeks, the foetus is approximately 6cm long. The eyelids are still shut, ears are forming and the brain is beginning to develop and grow. The internal sex organs are developing, but you can't tell the sex from the outside yet. The baby can curl its toes, absorb some nutrients through its digestive tract and swallow. Tiny nails are beginning to grow, the fingers and toes are no longer webbed and the eyes, nose, mouth and ears continue to develop. Twelve weeks is seen as an extremely significant watershed and traditionally marks the beginning of the second trimester. So we shall pick up on this journey of development in the next chapter.

CHINESE MEDICINE AND THE FIRST TRIMESTER

In the first trimester, you are building a lot of Blood for the foetus, which is produced by your digestion. So your digestive system is in overdrive during the first three months, often accompanied by pregnancy nausea because it is working so hard for your baby. I therefore recommend eating cooked foods, which are easier to digest than raw, and going for quality as much as possible when you don't feel like much in terms of quantity (see pp. 122–30 for nutrition during the first trimester). Raw foods tend to be Cold and therefore constricting, limiting the blood flow needed for the foetus.

At this time, you want to be bringing your Qi and blood to the centre, to your womb, so it is best to avoid pungent, strong-tasting foods during the first months of pregnancy, as these will tend to have a dispersing effect.

You might also experience cravings for particular foods – I urge my patients to listen to their cravings during pregnancy, as these often indicate something that you're lacking (see p. 131). Heightening your body awareness will also help you to address and even prevent some of the discomforting conditions of pregnancy. For example, you might feel warmed and comforted by ginger, but equally ginger might be too much heat and make you feel even worse. Don't persevere with foods that don't suit you; find instead the alternatives that work for your body.

If you can take it easy and rest as much as possible during the first trimester then the blood will flow to your uterus and to your digestion. Exercise takes blood to the limbs and muscles, which can put a strain on your digestion and weaken it during this important time. I know it's very easy to feel guilty about resting and, from a practical point of view, most of the people around you (including your work colleagues) won't even know you are pregnant at this stage. But the more you can rest and feel calm during the first trimester, the easier your entire pregnancy is likely to be. Your energy is being put to very good use as the embryo cells multiply at an amazing rate.

Sitting quietly, doing nothing, spring comes,
and the grass grows by itself.
Zen proverb

The old Chinese medicine texts advise avoiding sex and too much stimulation caused by passion, desires and overactivity. To be honest, I don't know many women who struggle with that advice, as sex is usually far from their minds (but don't think you are weird if you are still interested – just try not to get too overexcited!).

In the first two months, it is the baby's Jing that takes care of development – just as in Western medicine we talk about the 'foundations' of development and the 'blueprint' for the nervous system. So don't worry too much if you can't even hear the word 'vegetable' without feeling a wave of nausea at this stage. In most cases, pregnancy nausea tends to disappear in the second trimester and it is at that point that what you eat has much more of an impact on the health of your growing baby. This highlights the importance of a healthy pre-conception lifestyle which will pay some dividends now if all you can face is stodge.

I believe that a mother's experiences during pregnancy all have an impact on the growing baby. Even your innermost thoughts and feelings affect your baby; emotions have a vibration and it is that vibration that creates the baby's formative experiences and will shape its personality and spirit.

Pregnancy is the perfect time to rediscover all the things that make you feel good, as whatever has a positive effect on you also has a positive effect on your baby. Spend time with people who bring out good feelings in you; listen to your favourite music. If you have friends or colleagues who tend to stress you out, give yourself a bit of space from them around this time. It's a time to draw in as much energy as possible, especially calm and happy energy. In Chinese medicine, this time is described as 'the beginning of the education'[12] and 'the beginning of a person is the beginning of the heart/mind'.[13]

SUPER-DELUXE YOGA REST WITH YONI MUDRA

Lying on your yoga mat, use a pillow for your head and a bolster or two more pillows underneath your thighs and behind your knees. This eases off the curve in the lower back and brings a comforting tilt to the pelvis. Take two more pillows or cushions and place one under each elbow and upper arm. If the cushions feel too high, folded blankets may work better. The aim is for your elbows to be high enough to allow your hands to rest very comfortably over your belly. Let the thumb tips touch each other, resting just on or below the navel. Let the palms of the hands rest gently on the belly, with the index fingertips touching and the other fingertips pointing down towards the groin. This creates a downward pointing triangle which you can place over the womb, wherever you feel is most comfortable. This powerful hand gesture is called yoni mudra. (Yoni means 'the source' and, resting in this pose, you can take yourself back to your source of quiet rest and deep recuperation, while you feel the warmth of your hands nourishing your womb and your baby as she grows so rapidly within.)

Breathe freely and easily, close your eyes and enjoy the healing rest that comes with just being held and supported in this comfortable position. There is no need to move; simply being here and breathing freely is feeding you and your baby, re-energizing and revitalizing.

Whatever time you take to be in this resting pose will repay you in terms of renewed energy and a fresh perspective. Ideally, take half an hour or forty minutes, and while you are in the pose, listen to a relaxation CD (see recommendations on p. 343), or follow the instructions below:

- Settle your physical body. Feel the places where you have support from the floor, the pillows and, breathing out, deliver the weight of your body down into these supports. It is as if you give away the weight of your body, down into the earth. Breathe freely to settle the body.
- Mentally repeat your intention to gain the maximum benefits of this relaxation practice.
- Carry your mental attention around the physical body, greeting each part in turn.
- Breathe freely and easily.

- Return to your opening intention, repeat it again, then gradually and slowly reawaken the body. Stretch and wake up, perhaps using the womb greeting (see box below).

For more information on Uma Dinsmore-Tuli's books and website, and yoga in pregnancy, please see Resources, p. 339 and Further Reading, p. 347.

WOMB GREETING

Movement is not your top priority during the first trimester, but if you would like to add a simple gracious movement to the resting pose, then this womb greeting is a beauty.

Resting on your back, bend your knees so that the soles of your feet rest flat on the floor, about hip-distance apart. With your hands resting in yoni mudra (see p. 96) over your womb, ensure your elbows are well grounded either side of your hips – if the elbows touch the floor without the pillows or blankets beneath, you can remove the supports.

As you inhale, slowly spread the fingers and lift the forearms and hands, taking them up away from the womb and moving them out to the sides. At the end of the inhale, the backs of the hands rest on the floor.

As you exhale, slowly bring the palms of the hands back over to rest on your womb.

Match breath with movement, so that the rhythm of your breathing is synchronized with the opening and closing movement of the arms and hands over the womb. Repeat for nine breaths, or more, if you prefer.

Antenatal Check-ups and Tests

Between weeks 8 and 12 you will have the first of your antenatal check-ups, your 'booking appointment', and it's the perfect opportunity to ask your midwife or doctor any questions you may have or discuss any anxieties. This check-up will probably take a couple of hours. Your doctor will want to get to know your health background (similar to how we assess your Jing in Chinese medicine) and will give you a physical examination.

Health background
This will cover the following:

- ❀ Age
- ❀ Your general health and your partner's
- ❀ Date of your last period – to help calculate your due date
- ❀ Previous and/or current illnesses
- ❀ Previous pregnancy history, including any miscarriages
- ❀ Family history of inherited diseases and/or twins
- ❀ Ethnic origins (yours and your partner's, as some inherited diseases are more common in particular ethnic groups)
- ❀ Where you live, work and other general lifestyle questions
- ❀ How you are feeling

Physical examination
This will include a number of different checks, all of which are routine.

Height and weight
How much and how quickly you gain weight during your pregnancy can be useful signs for your midwife in terms of how your pregnancy is progressing and whether there might be any cause for concern. Your midwife will also help you with nutrition and diet advice to maintain healthy weight gain during pregnancy, as gaining far too much weight (or far too little) may be causes for concern when it comes to your baby's health. Information for eating well during the first trimester can be found on pp. 122–30.

Blood pressure
Your blood pressure will be taken at every antenatal check-up as it is a good indicator of how your body is coping with and adapting to pregnancy. Your doctor will also check your breathing and heart rate to get a good picture of your general health.

Urine sample

You'll probably be asked to bring a urine sample to all your antenatal check-ups. The main reason for this is to check for sugar in your urine; if you regularly have sugar present in your urine you may be at risk of developing gestational diabetes – a type of diabetes that disappears after pregnancy, but needs to be monitored and kept in check through diet (see p. 172) and occasionally requires insulin. Urine tests also check for proteins that may indicate either a urinary tract infection (see p. 113) or pre-eclampsia (see p. 221).

Blood sample

Your blood test will establish your blood type first of all, and check whether you are anaemic (see p. 134). You will also be checked for any diseases that could harm you or the baby.

HELPFUL INFORMATION

It's helpful to chat things through openly during this appointment, so that you feel as informed as possible and can then focus on all the positives. Your midwife or doctor should cover most questions as a matter of course, but it's handy to take a list with you as a reminder, in case you want to go through any specific areas. These might include:

- an overview of how the baby develops during pregnancy
- nutrition advice (see p. 102)
- general exercise advice (see p. 101)
- specific exercise questions (for example, whether you can go horse-riding)
- advice on pelvic-floor exercises (see p. 206)
- information on future antenatal screening tests, who will be caring for you, check-ups and classes
- an explanation of maternity benefits
- travel advice
- information on planning your labour, including where you want to have your baby (see p. 158).

Your midwife should take notes throughout this appointment and give a copy of them to you, along with lots of leaflets about various aspects of pregnancy, from nutrition to travel. Try to keep all your pregnancy notes together, so that you can easily find and refer to them, and also bring them along to future antenatal visits. You should also take your notes with you when travelling, so if you have any problems the local hospital (whether in the UK or abroad) will have details both of your antenatal care and the results of any investigations. You can also keep a note of any of the common conditions you experience through your pregnancy and what does or doesn't help.

AN INTEGRATED APPROACH

As you read through this book, you may decide you want to include some of the diet, exercise or emotional advice to help boost your well-being through pregnancy. You might choose to take a 'yoga for pregnancy' class or visit a qualified acupuncturist or osteopath or want to incorporate some of the techniques in the chapters on labour into your birth plan. Be open with your midwife and doctors about how you view your own health and pregnancy, as they are your primary healthcare providers and the information in this book is given very much in the spirit of being complementary. Communication is important, and I do regularly talk to midwives and obstetricians with a view to offering patients the best support. Expect your practitioners to do the same, as it is important to build this bridge.

Nuchal-fold test

You may be offered the nuchal-fold test, which screens for chromosomal abnormalities such as Down's syndrome. The test isn't a conclusive indicator one way or the other, but can indicate an increased likelihood of Down's syndrome earlier than a blood test (which would be done in Week 16, see p. 155). The nuchal-fold test is performed during an ultrasound scan and is often combined with a blood test (to measure two hormones – Beta HCG and PAPP A) to increase the detection rate. The nuchal fold is located at the back of the foetus's neck and is larger in babies with Down's syndrome, due to increased fluid retention in this area. The nuchal-translucency test will give an adjusted risk of Down's syndrome which should be compared with your age-related risk. If the risk is high, or you are concerned, the doctor should discuss the option of prenatal diagnostic tests (see p. 157).

Things to Avoid in Early Pregnancy

It is worthwhile being aware of things you need to avoid early on in your pregnancy.

Strenuous exercise and heavy lifting

In the early weeks of pregnancy, there is a risk that the fertilized egg can become detached from the uterine wall. Avoiding activities that use your abdominal muscles excessively, like stretching, very strenuous exercise and heavy lifting, is therefore advisable. Keep exercise very light; try gentle walks.

Smoking

The nicotine from smoking while pregnant goes through to the baby and smoking has been linked to a higher incidence of bleeding during pregnancy and miscarriage. Babies born to smokers tend to be smaller, more likely to suffer from breathing problems and may be less developed than babies born to non-smoking women. There are also links between a higher rate of cot death and babies born to mothers who smoke.

Breathing in someone else's smoke is also harmful, so it is best for partners to quit if they smoke, and for you to avoid second-hand smoke wherever possible.

Alcohol

Doctors have traditionally advised women to avoid drinking any alcohol during pregnancy. However, these guidelines have been changed to reflect research that suggests drinking up to a small glass of wine a day has no ill effects on the baby. It is still important to realize, however, that any alcohol you drink is passed through to the baby's bloodstream through the placenta, and that excessive drinking during pregnancy can lead to low birthweight and abnormalities.

X-rays

Any tests that use radiation may be harmful to your baby. Tell your GP if you had an X-ray or other form of test using radiation in the early weeks of pregnancy before you knew you were pregnant. Dentists often use X-rays, so you'll need to let them know you are pregnant.

Foods to avoid

Certain foods can contain harmful bacteria and so are best avoided. These include the following:

- ❀ Raw or partially cooked eggs
- ❀ Raw meat
- ❀ Liver and liver-based foods
- ❀ Pâtés
- ❀ Soft cheeses
- ❀ Potato salads and coleslaw
- ❀ Reheated foods, unless piping hot all the way through
- ❀ Unwashed fruit or vegetables
- ❀ Shark, swordfish or marlin
- ❀ Raw shellfish

Don't eat more than two portions of oily fish a week or four tins of tinned fish (for information visit www.eatingforpregnancy.org.uk). (See pp. 122–30 for nutrition during the first trimester.)

In addition to all of the above, the following should be avoided in early pregnancy:

- ❀ All essential oils
- ❀ All medications, unless cleared with your GP or obstetrician first
- ❀ Sunbeds

WARNING SIGNS DURING PREGNANCY

If you have any cause for concern about anything during your pregnancy, don't hesitate to discuss it with your doctor or midwife. Always go straight to your doctor if you experience any of the following warning signs:

- **Persistent vomiting** – where you are unable to tolerate fluids, or if nausea is accompanied by symptoms of dehydration (such as cracked lips or urinating only once or twice a day).
- **Severe abdominal pain** If you have not had a scan confirming a normal intra-uterine pregnancy, this may indicate ectopic pregnancy in the early months. Later in pregnancy, abdominal pain may indicate placental problems.
- **Any vaginal bleeding at any time during pregnancy** This doesn't necessarily mean that anything is wrong, but it is always best to check. It may indicate a miscarriage (see p. 148), especially in the first twelve weeks and if experienced alongside lower-back pain or cramps in the uterus. (See also 'Bleeding in Pregnancy' box, p. 106.)
- **Severe headaches** Headaches that don't go away or are experienced in your forehead area, intolerance to bright lights, and swelling in the hands and feet may indicate pregnancy-induced hypertension or pre-eclampsia.
- **Fever** Where there is a fever without cold or flu symptoms this may be an indication of infection.
- **A sudden increase in thirst** This may be a sign of developing gestational diabetes (see p. 172).
- **Itching** If you experience itching all over your body, this may indicate a serious condition called obstetric cholestasis (see p. 209).

PREVENTION IS BETTER THAN CURE

When Sally came to see me for her initial consultation, she was running ten minutes late and breathlessly rushed into the clinic, her energy bouncing off the walls. 'Sorry I'm late,' she gasped. 'I couldn't get out of the meeting on time, and then the trains were all delayed.'

Sally was in early pregnancy (eight weeks) and told me how it had taken some months to become pregnant. She was exhausted and feeling anxious about being pregnant. She had experienced some spotting (mild bleeding) and was really worried she might lose the baby.

Sally described her day to me, which started at six in the morning when she had a yogurt for breakfast before rushing to work in the city. Her journey was an hour, and she worked non-stop, occasionally with a break for lunch, until seven in the evening. She had been doing this for ten years. There were many computer screens in her office and she spent the whole day reading the markets from her computer. Her job was stressful and there was a culture of overwork in the office, with pressure on to be the first in and the last to leave. As a result, Sally usually got home at eight and slumped in front of the telly while her husband made her something to eat. She had very little appetite and no desire to cook or engage with her food. When her husband put a meal in front of her, she was able to eat it, but then felt exhausted soon afterwards. She told me that a few times she had become dizzy and faint on the Tube and had been really tearful.

Sally told me that she had begun to suffer from insomnia and would feel anxious at night, and although she was delighted about being pregnant, she had many fears about what it would bring. She had begun to suffer from palpitations and a feeling of impending doom. Her mother was unwell and she and her sister were taking turns to go and help out at weekends.

I got the feeling that Sally was hurtling at full speed towards a crisis; something needed to change, and it needed to change fast.

It is often very hard in these situations to tell someone that their life is completely out of sync. I am fully aware of the pressures that exist in some jobs to perform at the top level. Many women find it really hard to take a step back when they have worked so hard to achieve their position. However, there are times when health (and, in this case, the health of both the mother and the unborn child) is absolutely paramount.

What Chinese medicine is so good at is identifying the 'not-yet disease' – in other words the illness that is coming or likely to come. I felt this was just one of those times.

I asked Sally to consider the idea of taking a bit of time off work. I felt that if she took a step backwards she would be able to take a fresh look at the situation and reassess her priorities. I felt that from where she was sitting, it would be hard to make any real changes. It would also give her time to build some relaxation and calm into her busy life. I believe that although pregnancy is not an 'illness', it is really important to make space in your life for the baby. If you don't, it can hit you like a ton of bricks when the baby does arrive, and it is often women who enter motherhood exhausted from overwork who suffer from depression and anxiety in the postnatal period.

I gave Sally acupuncture that day with the intention of calming her mind and her Heart enough for her to make a good decision for herself. I chose points on the Heart channel and points to help her energy. I also picked points that I knew would help to give her mental clarity. As she lay there, I could sense that she was relaxing for the first time in a long time. Her breathing became deeper and the sense of calm around her was tangible.

I gave her no more advice that day. I said she was welcome to come back, but the most important decision she needed to make did not involve me giving her a long list of more things to do and to achieve. She could contact me whenever she wanted to.

Sally came back to see me a month later. She had reduced her working day and her employers had been much more understanding than she expected. Sally said she had got to the point where she was ready to walk away if it had come to it. She spoke about 'feeling clear about things for the first time in a while'. As soon as she had made the decision, she felt a great sense of relief, whatever the outcome at work.

Sally came regularly for treatment for several weeks and I saw her relax and change almost before my eyes. She slept better, she no longer felt anxious or tearful and her appetite returned. Although the treatments helped to focus her mind and to bring the body back towards normal function, it was the changes that she herself made that really made the difference.

Just before having the baby, Sally came back to see me for treatment. She told me how different she felt and how calm and grounded she felt about having her baby. She said she had intended to work right up until the birth, but had stopped a month before in order to rest and prepare herself for this next chapter in her life.

I could see that Sally had really stepped into her ability to make good decisions for herself. I felt that this was a vital lesson for her to take into motherhood and would serve her well in the future.

I have no doubt that if Sally had not changed her approach she would not have come out of it quite so well. I see a similar picture played out time and again in clinic, both in small ways and in life-changing ways, such as this case.

BLEEDING IN PREGNANCY

About a quarter of all women will experience mild spotting or even bleeding in early pregnancy. In most cases, this is considered completely normal, but it is important to always let your GP or midwife know if it is happening. It may occur around the time when your menstrual bleed would have been, or it can be part of the implantation process. In Chinese medicine, it is often a sign that the Spleen is weak and, as you know, the Spleen is all about digestion. One of the other things the Spleen does is to 'Hold the Blood'; so strengthening the Spleen through rest and good nutrition will go some way to helping with the spotting. If you are still exercising, maybe take it as a sign to cut back on this. Take the lift instead of the stairs (just for now), eat good, warm cooked food and go to bed early.

Common Conditions

Morning sickness (or pregnancy nausea)

The first thing to say about morning sickness is that its name is misleading: it does not only occur in the morning. Many a woman has complained to me, saying, 'What I have *can't* be *morning* sickness, because I feel sick the *entire* time!'

About half of all pregnant women experience nausea during their pregnancy, usually between weeks 6 and 16, but sometimes from as early as when their period would have been due and as late as right up to the birth. Often, there is respite during the second trimester, followed by reappearance in the last few weeks of pregnancy. But even women who don't feel nauseous often notice that their relationship with food is altered in some way. I think it's the body's way of asking us to simplify our diet at this stage.

Nausea and vomiting during pregnancy are not thought to affect the development of the foetus. However, the worry is that it might lead to dehydration. If your symptoms persist, and you can't keep anything down or begin to lose weight quickly, talk to your doctor.

Why does it happen?

From a Western perspective, there are different theories as to why women experience nausea during pregnancy. Dramatic changes to hormone levels, how the brain then reacts to those hormones, fatigue and stress levels and high emotions are all considered possible factors.

What can you do?

The NHS Choices website recommends making diet and lifestyle changes first and, if symptoms are persistent, your doctor may prescribe an anti-emetic (anti-sickness) medicine. Diet and lifestyle recommendations include getting plenty of rest, drinking and eating little and often, eating more savoury foods than sweet or spicy, eating plain biscuits before getting up (rich tea in bed first thing), avoiding foods or smells that trigger nausea and wearing comfortable clothes.

In Chinese medicine, we consider that pregnancy nausea (which I think is a more apt name) can manifest in several different ways and, like all things, 'the symptoms will determine the treatment'.

Tips for all

- ❀ Acupuncture can be very helpful in most cases[14], although sometimes treatment is required several times a week. I usually charge a reduced price in these situations; ask your acupuncturist for advice.
- ❀ Eat little and often, to prevent your blood-sugar levels from dropping, and simplify your diet.
- ❀ Be careful to avoid dehydration – simple soups are perfect.
- ❀ Try cutting out wheat.
- ❀ Sea sickness bands (available at most chemists) help, but the point can be hard to locate, so some women find they get no relief.
- ❀ Eat dry crackers before rising.
- ❀ Try taking 1 tablespoon of apple cider vinegar in hot water.
- ❀ Add one to two drops of peppermint oil to a bowl of boiling water – this will fill the air with a fresh smell, but don't stand directly over it or deeply inhale. Lemons are also helpful to add freshness to your environment.

Acupressure for pregnancy nausea

There are several points that you might find useful if you are suffering from nausea.

Kidney 6 (Kid 6)
Use this point whenever you feel queasy.

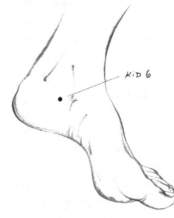

KID 6 IS A USEFUL POINT FOR ALL SICKNESS

KID 6

APPLY PRESSURE TO THE POINT (WHICH IS JUST BELOW THE BONE) WITH YOUR THUMB OR APPLY AN EAR-PRESS SEED TO WEAR ALL DAY

Pericardium 6 (P 6)

Apply pressure with thumbs or fingers until relief occurs.

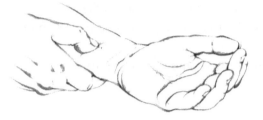

PL IS THE No. 1 POINT FOR NAUSEA

P6 IS THREE FINGERS' WIDTH ON THE INSIDE
OF THE FOREARM BETWEEN THE TWO TENDONS

Tips by type

Hot type

You are too hot in your Stomach and this makes the Stomach Qi rebel upwards. You will probably be vomiting after eating and have a strong thirst.

Tongue: Very red and/or with a yellow coating.

Tips: Eliminate all heating foods and add cooling foods into your diet (see chart, p. 59). Don't over-eat and drink fresh mint tea or chamomile tea. Do not eat or drink ginger.

Acupressure points: stimulate point St 44; the best way to do this is by squeezing it between thumb and forefinger.

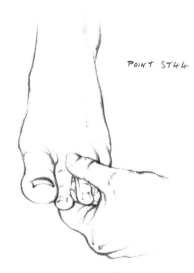

POINT ST44

THIS IS THE MAIN POINT TO USE
WHEN THE STOMACH IS TOO HOT; USE IN
SICKNESS AND IF YOU HAVE HEARTBURN

Phlegm type

If this is you, you will probably be carrying a tissue around with you trying to get rid of the excess saliva you are producing. You may well vomit and it will contain phlegm.

Tongue: A sticky coating and may look swollen.

Tips: Follow the diet to remove phlegm on p. 218 and make sure you don't become dehydrated.

Acupressure points: you should massage St 40.

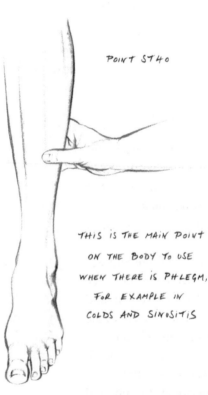

POINT ST 40

THIS IS THE MAIN POINT ON THE BODY TO USE WHEN THERE IS PHLEGM, FOR EXAMPLE IN COLDS AND SINUSITIS

Cold type

You will feel chilly and be feeling uncomfortable in the epigastric area (below the centre of the rib cage and above the belly button on the midline). When you vomit it will be clear fluid.

Tongue: Might have a white coating.

Tips: Listen to what your mum used to say and dress up warm; don't walk around with bare feet or midriff. Eat warming foods (see p. 58). Ginger is very good for you too,[15] although don't overdose or you may end up with Hot-type sickness.

Acupressure points: gently rub Ren 12 to generate warmth. You may find that this area even feels cold. If your tummy, or 'middle burner' as we say in Chinese medicine, is too cold, you need to warm it up.

REN 12 FOR MORNING SICKNESS

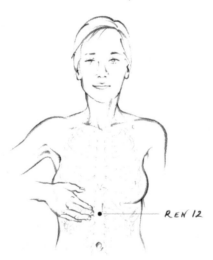

REN 12

GENTLY RUB REN 12 TO GENERATE WARMTH

Stagnant type

You are probably belching, and when you vomit it will be bitter and you will want to wash your mouth out. Your tummy probably looks more pregnant than you actually are (having fun yet?).

Tongue: Mauve with maybe some reddening on the sides.

Tips: If you are feeling anxious, stressed or conflicted about your pregnancy at all, all of which are very normal, relax as much as you can. It would be good to address any emotional issues that are plaguing you. Movement is also good – going for a walk and not sitting at your desk looking at a computer will help.

Acupressure points: Liv 3 (right), P 6 (see p. 109) – best stimulated by hooking the fingers under the foot and using the thumb to apply pressure to the point.

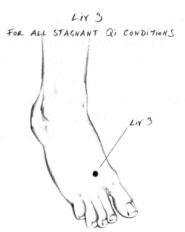

Liv 3
FOR ALL STAGNANT Qi CONDITIONS

Liv 3

LIV 3 IS A GREAT POINT FOR WHEN THINGS ARE STUCK; IT'S ALSO USEFUL FOR OVERCOMING IRRITABLE MOOD

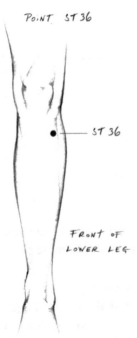

POINT ST 36

ST 36

FRONT OF LOWER LEG

ST 36 IS THE MAIN POINT FOR IMPROVING ENERGY LEVELS AND BUILDING Qi

Weak type

You can hardly pull yourself out of bed, every limb feels heavy and tired and you have no appetite. Your voice has shrunk and everything is an effort. You feel sick towards the end of the day, and feel drained by vomiting. *Tongue:* Pale and flabby.

Tips: You need to conserve your energy and eat little and often. You may not feel like eating, but actually it will make you feel better. Rest and you will begin to build more energy.

Acupressure points: St 36 (left) and Ren 12 (see p. 111)

Reflexology for pregnancy nausea

Massaging the entire web area between the thumb and forefinger with a 'cater-pillar' technique (see p. 335), helps to return the healing energy to the whole stomach area and encourage a normal functioning. Continue until you've covered the webbing, rather like the spokes of a wheel. Work for two minutes.

Urinary-tract infection (UTI)

Often also referred to as cystitis, this condition involves burning, painful and frequent urination.

Why does it happen?

Because the hormones of pregnancy make the muscles relax, the uterus enlarges and applies pressure on the bladder. The urethra may also relax, increasing the chance of ascending infection. If left untreated, it may progress into a kidney infection (pyelonephritis) which requires medical attention. Pyelonephritis may increase the risk of early labour. Signs of kidney infection include lower-back or tummy ache, fever and frequent urination.

What can you do?

As soon as you experience the early signs of a possible urinary tract infection (UTI) tell your midwife or doctor as it is important this condition is carefully monitored. It can become more serious and quite quickly too. The advice below should not take the place of medical guidance, but it can be helpful, especially if you are mindful and catch this very early.

Tips for all

- ❀ Drink plenty of water, a litre bottle, the minute you think you may be developing a urinary problem.
- ❀ Drink barley water (see p. 215 for recipe).
- ❀ Avoid sugar.
- ❀ Drink cranberry juice (if you can find it without sugar).
- ❀ Nettle tea is a great tonic (especially in the final trimester as it strengthens the Kidney energy).
- ❀ Dandelion leaves have a cooling and bitter nature that clear the burning sensation from a UTI and help urination. Pumpkin seeds

have also been used to benefit the bladder. Try dandelion leaf salad with slices of pear and a sprinkling of pumpkin seeds (season with olive oil and basil).

❀ Finely chop fresh dandelion root with some nettle leaf and boil for twenty minutes in water. Strain and drink.
❀ Avoid eating hot and spicy foods.
❀ The traditional remedy of drinking bicarbonate of soda with water should be avoided during pregnancy due its high salt content, which can increase blood pressure and lead to fluid retention.

Personal hygiene

❀ Wipe front to back after bowel movements and do not use any perfumed wipes or products anywhere near your vagina.
❀ No bubble baths, salts or soap in the bath.
❀ Always urinate after sex.
❀ Change out of wet swimsuits.

Useful point Kid 3 (Kidney 3)

This is a very good acupressure point if you are suffering from cystitis.

KID 3 IS A GREAT POINT FOR
WHEN YOU FEEL TIRED TO THE BONE

IT'S ALSO A GOOD POINT FOR URINARY CONDITIONS
AND BACK PROBLEMS

Tips by type
Cold type
Increased desire to urinate but no burning. Dragging-down feeling with urine flow that feels like it is finished, but then dribbles again. You may also experience lower-back ache and feel tired.

Tongue: Pale and/or swollen.

Tips: Introduce some warming foods and eliminate cold foods. Warming foods include oats, rice, squash, cherry, date, salmon and chicken (see p. 59 for cold foods to avoid).

Hot type
Dark urine and not much of it, pain and restlessness. You might be having trouble sleeping and be feeling thirsty.

Tongue: Red, sometimes with an even redder tip.

Tips: Introduce Heat-clearing foods and add some cooling ones, including apple, banana, barley, lemon and cucumber.

Damp type
Cloudy urine with a strong smell, burning sensation with a thirst, but strangely no desire to drink.

Tongue: Red prickles and a yellow coating.

Tips: Introduce foods to clear Dampness, including adzuki beans, jasmine tea, lemon and pumpkin and stay clear of foods that cause Dampness (see p. 225). Do not sit around in damp swimsuits; if you are on holiday, always change into a dry suit after swimming. I cannot tell you how often I give this advice to pregnant women, and although it seems old-fashioned it works a treat.

Tiredness and exhaustion
This is one of the most common complaints I get in clinic. Tiredness can tell the acupuncturist a great deal – we are in the realms of Qi here and this is our territory. So the good news is, there is much that I can do to help improve a pregnant woman's energy and much that you can do yourself.

A simple rule of tiredness in pregnancy when trying to understand Qi is to ask yourself these two questions:

❀ 'Do I feel better when I rest?' If so, you are deficient (lacking) in energy and you need to rest more.

❀ 'Do I feel better for movement?' If so, you are Stagnant and you need to move more (but do not overexert yourself or you will end up deficient).

Why does it happen?

Much of tiredness in the first trimester is due to the enormous number of changes your body is going through. Hormones are changing rapidly and the placenta which will keep your baby alive is forming. High levels of progesterone during the first trimester can have a sedative effect. If you need to get up and go to the loo a lot more during the night, you'll start to lose out on your usual deep sleep, and if you are suffering from pregnancy nausea and sickness, this too can sap your energy and leave you feeling drained.

Tiredness can also be a sign that you are developing anaemia, especially if you have other symptoms such as dizziness, fainting, shortness of breath or palpitations (see p. 134). If people comment that you are looking pale, you should keep an eye on your symptoms. Apart from meaning that you are not feeling at or anywhere near your best, anaemia can make you more prone to infection, early delivery and haemorrhages. This is why your midwife will want to test your blood and may prescribe iron supplementation.

What can you do?

Don't fight through your tiredness, take it as a sign that you need to rest. Start building rest times into your day now, as your life and your body make their shift towards motherhood. And try to use your evenings for putting your feet up; see people at weekends, rather than trying to fit too much in during the week.

This isn't a prescription for you to be in bed by eight from now until you're ready to give birth, but just until your energy levels recover.

Tips for all

❀ If you work and are struggling with early pregnancy tiredness then try to have a rest at lunchtime and put your health ahead of working long hours.

✿ Ask your partner to help out as much as possible with things like cooking and cleaning.

✿ If you already have young children, try to grab a nap when they do, rather than using the time as a whirlwind hour of washing, ironing and catching up with emails.

Tips by type

Tiredness and Blood Deficiency

You will feel like the energy has been drained out of you by a blood-sucking vampire and you will be looking like a member of the cast of *Twilight*! You will be pale, listless, have minimal enthusiasm and want to do as little as possible. You may feel faint or dizzy, with floaters in your field of vision. Anxiety is likely, which may interrupt your sleep, and you might even have palpitations.

Tongue: Pale sides.

Tips: • Moxibustion is great for this on St 36 (see p. 333). Try it every day for ten minutes – it will help to strengthen your body and your digestion to make plenty of blood.

• Include plenty of Blood-nourishing foods in your diet (see p. 57).

• Sprinkle black sesame seeds on steamed leafy greens and eat plenty of chicken soup (see recipe, p. 314). Kidney beans are also excellent, and apricots after food will help with iron absorption. Try my apricot flapjacks (see recipe, p. 120).

• Go to bed early and don't overdo the exercise.

• Build an element of rest into your day between 1 and 3 p.m., even if it is just laying your head on your desk for forty winks; you need to disengage your brain from work for a period of time to recharge.

Tiredness and Yang Deficiency

This is usually the sort of tiredness that is accompanied by a feeling of coldness. There is a sluggish, heavy feeling and everything feels slow. Even the slightest activity leaves you feeling worn out and it gets worse as the day progresses. It can affect the Spleen (digestion), the Heart (emotions) or the Kidneys (lower-back ache and coldness).

Tongue: Typically, it will look large because it is swollen.

Tips: • No raw or Cold foods (p. 59) or cold (temperature) drinks.
  • Try moxibustion to warm St 36 (see p. 333).
  • If you have a cold lower back with aching, then moxibustion or a hot-water bottle on your back will feel wonderful.
  • Include foods to nourish the Spleen like squash, chestnuts, garlic and warming spices (ginger, cardamom and cloves).
  • If you are physically working hard, take a few steps back.
  • Dress up warm.
  • Don't swim for now until your energy improves, as your body needs heating.

Tiredness and Yin Deficiency

Although you are tired, you also feel agitated and restless and just can't seem to switch off. Meditation and yoga are the last things on your mind, even though you sense they would help you. You might have night sweats and feel feverish in the afternoon at work.

Tongue: Crimson with a patch that looks as though it has been peeled or scraped off.

Tips: • As hard as you might find it, you need to find ways to switch off mentally. You will struggle later on if you don't learn this skill, and this is the typical picture of a very anxious mum! You crave stimulation but you need to unwind, and no one is going to help you with this except you. Try to avoid computers in the evening, or phones, or even the television. Find a way to build in downtime; if you can't face a yoga class, lie on your bed for half an hour when you get back from work, light a candle and put on a meditation CD – you are going to need to learn how to relax, so there is no better time than now.
  • Avoid stimulants in your food as well; coffee is off the menu, I'm afraid, and anything else with caffeine in it.
  • Try my fish and coconut curry recipe (see p. 121).
  • Eat little and often and avoid sugars. Tropical fruits are great for you – pineapple, mango, coconut, papaya and banana are all good for nourishing the Yin. Make a smoothie in the morning and add some linseeds (see p. 241).

Tiredness and Stagnation

Although this tends to kick in during the third trimester, as it becomes harder to move around, it can happen at any time in pregnancy, especially if you were a bit of a gym bunny prior to conceiving and have had to slow down. Generally, you will feel better for movement and a brisk walk in the fresh air. Your body might feel stiff and tight. There is often an emotional component to this type of tiredness: frustration, irritability, depression. You might sigh a lot.

I often see this pattern in women who have worked out regularly in the gym as a way to keep fit and slim, but who also use exercise to help with their mood. When they are unable to keep this up, the body finds it hard to move Qi around effectively. Sometimes, if you can make a mental swing to embrace gentler forms of exercise, then you'll shift the Stagnation. Swimming or walking, for example, are much more appropriate forms of exercise than running.

If you feel that you have unresolved emotional issues, now is the time to look into what you might be able to do to help yourself. It may be that the methods offered in this book are enough to help you through, or you may feel you need more professional help (see Resources, p. 339).

Tongue: Mauve-coloured.

Tips: Move around more; try not to sit at your desk all day without regular movement and walks. Stretching and yoga will help with tight muscles and stiffness.

Apricot and Toasted Pumpkin Seed Flapjacks

Apricots nourish blood and pumpkin seeds drain dampness (counteract dampening effect of sugar)

Makes about 12

50g (1¾oz) raw unsalted pumpkin seeds
170g (6oz) butter
20g (¾oz) agave or golden syrup
250g (9oz) porridge oats
50g (1¾oz) dried apricots, diced
125g (4½oz) brown sugar
pinch of sea salt

1. Preheat the oven to 180°/350°F/gas mark 4 and grease an 18 x 28cm (7 x 11in) Swiss roll tin.
2. In a frying pan, over medium–high heat, toast the pumpkin seeds for 5 minutes or so, until they are lightly browned. Remove from the heat and set aside to cool.
3. In a medium-sized saucepan, melt the butter and syrup together, then add the toasted seeds and all the remaining ingredients.
4. Pour the flapjack mixture into the prepared baking tin and spread evenly. Bake for 15–20 minutes until golden brown and firm to the touch.
5. Remove from the oven and let the flapjacks sit for 10 minutes, before cutting into squares and removing from the tin with a spatula.

Fish with a Coconut Curry Sauce

Perfect Yin/Yan balance: the cooling qualities of white fish and coconut with the heating spices of chillies

Serves 4–6

olive oil for cooking

2.5cm (1in) piece fresh ginger root, peeled and chopped into matchsticks

2 yellow onions, sliced thinly

4 garlic cloves, peeled and finely chopped

4 tomatoes, cored, peeled and chopped

2 teaspoons organic curry powder mix (or mix ground fenugreek, turmeric, cloves, coriander, cumin and ginger)

½ teaspoon ground cumin

1 teaspoon sea salt

½ teaspoon red chilli pepper flakes (optional)

freshly ground black pepper

small bunch fresh coriander, leaves only

300ml (10fl oz) coconut milk

600g (1lb 5oz) fish fillets (salmon, cod or halibut), cut into 3cm (1¼in) strips

1. Preheat the oven to 180°C/350°F/gas mark 4.
2. Add a couple of glugs of olive oil to a large saucepan with a lid (suitable for the oven), over medium–high heat. Add the fresh ginger, onions and garlic and sauté for a few minutes.
3. Add the tomatoes, and stir well. (You want the tomatoes to become mushy in the sauce.) Add the curry powder, cumin, salt, chilli flakes, black pepper and half of the fresh coriander leaves. Stir well.
4. Add the coconut milk and simmer for 5–10 minutes, so all the flavours start to blend together.
5. Add the fish strips, stirring in gently, then put the lid on the saucepan and transfer to the preheated oven. Bake for about 20 minutes, until the fish is cooked through.
6. Remove from the oven and taste for seasoning. Sprinkle with the rest of the coriander leaves before serving with jasmine rice for a deliciously hearty, nourishing meal.

Is the Fuel Good?

Eating well is helpful during the first trimester, but is not the be-all and end-all if you are struggling with nausea. There is plenty of time to catch up and the best advice is to try and eat a simple and nourishing diet of foods that are easy to digest.

Just think of the growth and development that happens in the nine months of pregnancy. Through your diet, your baby will receive all the nutrition needed to form organs, circulatory, digestive and other systems, the senses of smell, sight, taste and hearing. Eating well is also linked to healthy birthweight; babies who are born too small are more likely to have health problems and babies who are too big can complicate delivery, making intervention more likely.

Food can play a helpful role in alleviating, even preventing, certain common conditions in pregnancy: a diet with a healthy balance of complex carbohydrates, like oats and rice, can help reduce fatigue; one rich in fibre can relieve (or even prevent) constipation; while adopting the 'little and often' mantra can help prevent both nausea and heartburn.

In Chinese medicine, eating well during pregnancy is also vital as the digestion plays such an important role in building the Blood for the foetus. During pregnancy, we focus on particular nourishing types of food, especially Blood-nourishing and warming foods. We look to gently strengthen the Spleen and avoid foods that tend to increase Dampness, which often occurs with pregnancy. Suggestions are very similar to those of healthy eating in general, with a few added:

- ✿ Eat well, eat light – little and often – and don't skip meals.
- ✿ Eat seasonal foods.
- ✿ Eat slowly and chew properly to aid digestion.
- ✿ Don't eat late at night.
- ✿ Eat organic food, where possible.
- ✿ In Chinese medicine, the stomach digests both thought and food – so try not to watch TV, study or read while you are eating, as this will take energy away from the food being digested efficiently.
- ✿ Always eat a good breakfast if you can.

- ❀ Drink when you feel thirsty – don't flood your system to meet a quota.
- ❀ Eat warming foods (see below).
- ❀ Eat more cooked foods and fewer raw ones.
- ❀ Avoid pungent foods (see p. 124).
- ❀ Understand your cravings (see p. 131).

Store cupboard for the first trimester

The following food lists are simply some foods that are considered to be especially beneficial. So long as you are eating as healthily as you can, which isn't always easy during the first trimester with pregnancy nausea to contend with, you'll be doing a great job on the fuel front. The message really is to eat what you can and not to worry if that often means a few dry crackers and a bit of chicken soup.

For all

- ❀ Grains: oats, rice
- ❀ Vegetables: carrots, kale, pumpkin, squash, oyster, reishi and shiitake mushrooms
- ❀ Fruit: blackberries, cherries, dates, figs, grapes, papaya
- ❀ Pulses: adzuki beans, chickpeas, lentils, tempeh
- ❀ Nuts and seeds: almonds, coconut, hazelnuts, sunflower seeds
- ❀ Fish: herring, salmon, tuna, mackerel, sardines (limit to two portions a week)
- ❀ Meat/dairy: chicken, ham, quail, turkey, egg white
- ❀ Herbs and spices: liquorice
- ❀ Condiments: olive oil, miso, molasses, brown sugar

Warming foods

Throughout pregnancy, it is a good idea to eat warming foods, unless you show specific signs of Heat like a strong thirst, redness in the eyes, lack of urine and dry stools, and may need more neutral and cooling foods to help create a good balance.

How you cook foods has an effect on their temperature, and stewing or stir-frying are both particularly warming ways of cooking. You can also begin to tell the temperature of foods by how they grow: plants which take longer to grow, like root vegetables and ginger, tend to be more warming than fast-growing vegetables like lettuce and courgettes. And foods with higher water content, like cucumber and melon, tend to be more cooling.

Warming foods include pumpkin, squash, reishi mushrooms, cherries, black beans, tempeh, chestnuts, coconut, salmon, chicken, pheasant, turkey, milk, hawthorn, miso, molasses and brown sugar. Ginger, well known for helping many women with pregnancy nausea, is described in Chinese medicine as a Hot food, and so can be a little overwhelming for some constitutions. Be aware of how different foods make you feel.

Avoiding pungent foods

Most herbs and spices are 'pungent' foods and it can be helpful to avoid these during the first trimester to give your digestion a helping hand. Similarly, Western advice will often be to eat slightly more bland and naturally sweeter foods like carrots and squash, as opposed to strong-tasting dark green leafy vegetables.

Avoiding Dampness

Here in the UK, we are often prone to Dampness because of our climate, our Western diet and lifestyle. With my patients, I often see the signs of Dampness materialize in conditions like oedema (see p. 211) or sinusitis (see p. 216) or catching a cold and finding it impossible to shift. Eating little and often, avoiding too much raw or rich, fatty or overly sweet food are all good ways to avoid Dampness. Specific foods which are helpful include adzuki beans, barley, jasmine tea, marjoram, onion, parsley and pumpkin.

Ideas for meals

Where I have suggested a salad, eat it with a soup on all but the warmest of summer days.

Blood-nourishing

❀ Leafy green salad with watercress, avocado and hard-boiled egg; eat with a miso soup
❀ Chicken casserole

- ❀ Mushroom lasagne
- ❀ Beetroot soup
- ❀ Spinach omelette
- ❀ Snacks: grapes, dates, figs, apricots, apples, almonds
- ❀ Tea: nettle

Qi-nourishing

- ❀ Stir-fried chicken with mushroom and asparagus
- ❀ Cottage pie
- ❀ Baked sweet potato
- ❀ Aubergine – oven-baked with tahini, garlic, lemon and pomegranate seeds (see below)
- ❀ Oily fish: herring, mackerel, tuna, sardines (limit to two portions a week)
- ❀ Snacks: oat flapjack with honey and dates, grapes, cherries, dates, figs, almonds, walnuts
- ❀ Tea: liquorice

Aubergine and Pomegranate Salad with Lemon Tahini Dressing
Aubergine moves stagnant blood

Serves 4

For the tahini:
170g (6oz) sesame seeds
1/3 teaspoon sea salt
60ml (2fl oz) walnut oil

For the dressing:
80ml (3fl oz) lemon juice
80ml (3fl oz) olive oil
90g (3oz) tahini
1/3 teaspoon sea salt
1/3 teaspoon cayenne pepper

For the salad:
1 medium–large aubergine
olive oil, for drizzling
freshly ground black pepper
1 medium–large pomegranate
1 small bunch coriander – leaves only
100g (3½oz) feta cheese

1. Preheat the oven to 180°C/350°F/gas mark 4.
2. To make the tahini, spread the sesame seeds in a thin layer on a baking sheet and bake for 10 minutes, until golden brown. Remove from the oven and set aside to cool. When cool, blend in a high-speed blender with the salt, slowly adding the walnut oil, until you have a smooth paste. This makes double the amount needed for the recipe.
3. Increase the oven temperature to 200–220°C/400–425°F/gas mark 6–7. Slice the aubergine into 1cm (½in) slices and lay them flat in one or two oven dishes. Drizzle each piece with olive oil and grind some black pepper over them. Turn them over and repeat this process, then turn them another couple of times and drizzle with more oil, so it's nicely absorbed. Bake for 45 minutes, turning 3 or 4 times during cooking, so that each piece gets well browned. Remove from the oven and set aside to cool.
4. Deseed the pomegranate and set aside.
5. To make the dressing, blend the lemon juice, olive oil, and tahini with the salt and cayenne pepper and 2 tablespoons of water until emulsified. (This makes double the amount of dressing needed. The remainder can be stored in the fridge in an airtight container for a week or so.)
6. When the aubergine slices have cooled, place them on a serving dish and sprinkle with the pomegranate seeds and coriander leaves. Slice the feta thinly and dot pieces all over the salad. Spoon the dressing over the top and serve immediately.

Vitamins and minerals

There are certain vitamins, minerals and food groups that you need more of during pregnancy. In Chinese medicine, we don't think in terms of vitamin A or C as such, but the understanding of how certain foods help the body is similar, so I think these are helpful to include. Your prenatal supplement will include a good supply of the vitamins you need, but you'll gain even more benefit from natural food sources.

Vitamin A

Needed for the growth and development of cells, bones, eyes, skin, teeth and immunity. It is important not to have too much vitamin A in the diet, so liver and liver-based foods are to be avoided during pregnancy (see p. 102 for a comprehensive list of foods to avoid).

Sources of vitamin A include dairy foods, green leafy vegetables, carrots, pumpkin, squash, red peppers, whole grains (including oats), mangoes, apricots.

Vitamin B1

Essential for converting carbohydrates into energy, this vitamin also helps to promote appetite, so it can help a great deal with tiredness during pregnancy. It promotes the production of red blood cells for the baby.

Sources of vitamin B1 include oats, peas, raisins, cauliflower, nuts, corn and sunflower seeds.

Vitamin B2

This helps your body to release energy from fats and proteins as well as carbohydrates. For the baby, vitamin B2 aids cell division and tissue growth and repair. (In the third trimester, in particular, it helps with brain growth.) A deficiency of this vitamin can cause poor bone formation, poor digestion and a suppressed immune system in the foetus.

Sources of vitamin B2 include chicken, milk, yogurt, eggs, mushrooms and peas.

Vitamin B3

Another B vitamin that helps to release energy from food, this also increases circulation and blood flow, so improving the flow of nutrients to the baby.

Too much vitamin B3 can cause itchy skin and also stomach problems. Sources of vitamin B3 include fish, chicken, lamb and mushrooms.

Vitamin B6

This helps to build tissue and red and white blood cells, and affects the proteins specific to the brain and nervous system. It is also thought this vitamin may help with pregnancy nausea.

Sources of vitamin B6 include bananas, avocado, bran, meat, potatoes and spinach.

Vitamin B7

This vitamin is needed for DNA replication as the foetus cells divide, and for digesting fats, carbohydrates and proteins. Insufficient B7 can trigger fatigue, nausea, muscle pain and skin problems.

Sources of vitamin B7 include bananas, nuts, eggs and whole grains.

Vitamin B12

B12 partners with folate (folic acid) to aid healthy development, so deficiencies can cause neural-tube defects, including spina bifida and digestive disorders.

The only natural dietary sources of vitamin B12 are animal products, including meat, eggs, dairy and fish. If you are a vegan, you'll need to get your B12 from supplements.

Choline

Another B family member, choline helps with brain development, including learning and memory.

Sources of choline include eggs, cauliflower, soybeans and meat.

Folic acid

Another B vitamin, folic acid is the one you are most likely to know about in relation to pregnancy. It is during the first trimester that the baby's brain and nervous system develop, and low levels of folic acid in the early months of pregnancy have been shown to cause around 70 per cent of all neural-tube defects. Folic acid also helps to produce red blood cells, encourages healthy birthweight and is associated with a lowered risk of premature birth. A deficiency can also trigger anaemia (see p. 134) in the mother, causing even more exhaustion.

Take 400mcg (0.4mg) folic acid supplements every day for the first twelve weeks of your pregnancy. If you are at high risk of having a baby born with a neural-tube defect (NTD), your doctor will prescribe a higher dose.

Sources of folic acid include bananas, avocados, green leafy vegetables, fruit and lentils.

Vitamin C
This vitamin produces collagen – the protein essential for the baby's developing cartilage, muscles, blood vessels and bones. Vitamin C helps in the absorption of iron and may also help you resist infection. Deficiencies may lead to a higher risk of pre-eclampsia later in pregnancy (see p. 221) and premature labour.

Sources of vitamin C include lemon, broccoli, kale, cabbage, peppers, tomatoes, berries, mangoes and melon.
Note: Orange juice is very Heating (and acidic), so in terms of colds and flu I would recommend that you avoid it. Also avoid it if you are suffering from any acid heartburn.

Vitamin D
This helps in the absorption of calcium and is, therefore, essential for developing bones and teeth.

Sources of vitamin D include sunlight, sardines and egg yolks.

Vitamin K
Essential for blood clotting, this can also help prevent excess blood loss after childbirth.

Sources of vitamin K include rapeseed oil, olive oil, avocado, oats and bananas.

Calcium
You probably know calcium is good for strong bones and teeth, but it is also needed for blood clotting, normal heart rhythm, nerve development and muscle contraction.

Sources of calcium include milk and other dairy foods, tofu, almonds, green leafy vegetables, broccoli and sardines.

Iron

Iron is vital in the production of red blood cells and distributing oxygen around the body, but many women find it a challenge to get enough iron into their diet, especially during pregnancy when blood production steps up three gears. A deficiency in iron may lead to low birthweight or a premature baby, as well as fatigue and eventually anaemia in the mother. But be aware that too much iron can cause constipation (see p. 240).

Sources of iron include red meat, spinach and other dark green leafy vegetables, lentils and oats.

Magnesium

Magnesium works with calcium to help with developing bones and teeth, as well as with nerve and muscle function. It is also needed for regulating blood-sugar levels and in the removal of toxins from the body. Magnesium relaxes muscles, and so can help with leg cramps (see p. 191) and constipation (see p. 240).

Sources of magnesium include nuts, beans, tofu, natural yogurt, prunes and leafy vegetables.

Zinc

There has been much research into zinc and pregnancy, which suggests that insufficient zinc may increase the risk of miscarriage, low birthweight and premature delivery. Zinc is also essential for growth, from early cell division to bones, hair and skin.

Sources of zinc include beef, turkey, natural yogurt, oats and eggs.

Weight gain

We are a society fixated on diets, some healthy, some obsessive. So the thought of 'healthy weight gain' sends some pregnant women into panic mode. If you are feeling anxious about gaining weight, read the section on worry (p. 139) and think of how pregnancy gives you the perfect opportunity to relax about your relationship with food and focus on health.

Your doctor or midwife will probably recommend your ideal weight gain, based on factors such as your height, weight and resulting BMI (body mass index). If your weight is average, your suggested weight gain will likely be between 11.25 and 16kg (25 and 35lb). If you are below or above average, your ideal weight gain may be a little more or less than the average, more if you are underweight and less if you are overweight. Although the common figure for the amount of extra calories you need is 300 during the second and third trimester, you need fewer during the first. The key, though, is to listen to your body, rather than religiously counting calories. If you are gradually gaining weight without sudden jumps then you're on the right track.

In the first trimester most women need to gain about 900g–1.8kg (2–4lb), so not much. Weight gain should then pick up quite considerably during the second trimester, then slow down again in the third. In the ninth month, weight gain often stops altogether for some women; every pregnancy is different.

Cravings . . .

Most women experience food cravings at some point during pregnancy, usually in the first trimester. Sweet flavours, dairy and salty foods are the most common cravings, often in unusual combinations. It's no wonder that you might crave sweetness as sweet foods nourish the Spleen, which needs to be working well during pregnancy, helping the digestion to produce extra Blood for your developing baby. The thing is, when our bodies crave sweet foods, berries or a carrot are what it's really after, but it's so much easier to reach for a doughnut or a bar of chocolate. Likewise, your body might signal a craving for sodium in the form of salty foods, but will need only a little to redress the balance; or a craving for fatty takeaways might actually signpost a need for more high-quality fats in the diet. Foods that are processed or manufactured tend to be at the extremes – very sweet, rich or salty. Don't worry or feel guilty if you devour the odd piece of chocolate cake, but if you can reach for natural food equivalents, you'll comfort your cravings without going too far in the opposite nutritional direction.

Here are some tips to help with your cravings:

❀ Eating a good breakfast can keep cravings in check.
❀ Listen to your cravings and think about whether you could make the odd healthy substitution.

❀ Have a little of what you fancy instead of a lot, and see if that does the trick.

❀ If you crave anything inedible like clay or ashes (a condition called pica), this could indicate a mineral deficiency. Always tell your doctor straight away and never give in to these cravings.

SOPHIE DAHL'S CRAVING FOR PINEAPPLE

'The moment I became pregnant I *longed* for pineapple. Ached for it. I've never been a particular pineapple fiend, but clearly I craved something it offered. This carried on and I would obsess about it at 3 a.m. I am told by Emma, the goddess of all things fertile, that pineapple is one of the few fruits that doesn't have an excessively dampening effect in small doses, offering instead a decongestant effect, which is particularly beneficial during the second trimester.

I suggest making double batches of this so you can have it close at hand.'

Pineapple and Mint Granita

Makes around 500ml (18fl oz)
2 pineapples, skin removed and cut into chunks (you can use bought
    pineapple juice if you like, but fresh pineapple is pretty spectacular)
2 sprigs of mint
agave to sweeten (optional)

1. Place the pineapple chunks in the food processor and whizz until you have mostly juice. Strain through a fine sieve.
2. In a heatproof bowl, blanch the mint sprigs with a little boiling water, then remove and run immediately under ice-cold water. Chop the mint finely and stir into the strained pineapple juice. Taste for sweetness and add agave if needed.

3. Freeze in a shallow metal container for around 2 hours. Check on it, and use a fork to break up what should be shards of icy pineapple mixture. Refreeze for a few hours. Using a fork, shave the crushed pineapple mixture into glasses and serve, or like me, eat it from the container, in bed.

Note from Emma: On the hottest of days, I think this would be delicious made with watermelon, which is great for keeping blood pressure down.

. . . and food aversions

As with cravings, well over three quarters of women experience food aversions during pregnancy. Some researchers say that both aversions and cravings are down to your hormones, as they peak during the greatest period of hormonal changes and tend to pass by the time you are halfway through your pregnancy. Others believe that they are an in-built instinct that steers pregnant women away from pungent foods (which, thousands of years ago, meant toxic plants) and towards sweeter grains and fruits.

Here are some tips for food aversions:

❀ Stick with mild-tasting, mild-smelling foods.
❀ Don't fight your aversions. If you're worried about not getting enough vitamins or nutrients, check out the store-cupboard foods on p. 123 for lots of alternatives; but it's OK if all you can manage is a bit of chicken soup and rice – that and your prenatal supplement should provide all the absolute essentials during the early months.
❀ If you are struggling with green vegetables, try orange instead, including carrots, pumpkin and squash.

YOUR SENSE OF SMELL

Most women experience a heightened sense of smell while pregnant, thanks, again, to hormones. I remember when I was pregnant even the chemicals used in magazine production used to send my head spinning. We can't prove it one way or the other, but perhaps this was Mother Nature's way of helping out, so that women would steer clear of strong-smelling and potentially sickness-inducing foods.

You might feel better swapping to mild, natural toiletries, washing your clothes more often and with mild detergent, opening the windows if cooking creates a smell and avoiding, wherever possible, any smells that make you feel queasy. Natural aromas that pregnant women seem to feel better with include lemon, mint and, for some women more than others, ginger.

Common Conditions

Anaemia

Oxygen is transported through the body by haemoglobin in red blood cells. Anaemia occurs when there is not enough haemoglobin within the blood, and may result in tiredness, breathlessness, palpitations and looking pale. It can also lead to an increase in infections.

Why does it happen?

There are two types of anaemia: iron-deficiency anaemia (most common) and pernicious anaemia.

Iron-deficiency anaemia

This is usually caused either by a diet that lacks the foods which will provide a good source of iron or from a digestive system that has poor absorption. Vitamin C, folic acid, B6 and B12 are all essential for iron absorption. This type of anaemia can also tend to occur at around twenty weeks when there is an increase in the woman's blood volume and also in the last four weeks. But it may occur at any time during pregnancy.

Pernicious anaemia

This may be caused either through a diet which is lacking in vitamin B12 or from a stomach problem which inhibits the absorption of B12. Treatment may involve B12 supplements (orally or by injection).

BE GOOD TO YOUR LIVER

There is a strong relationship between the Blood and the Liver, so whenever there is a problem or imbalance with the Blood, it is necessary to address the Liver. On an emotional level, the Liver gives us a sense of direction and the ability to envision our future – perhaps a good thing to consider when bringing a new life into the world.

Start the day with a cup of hot water and a slice of lemon or cider vinegar and a little honey.

Eat plenty of:

- green foods like seaweed, spinach and leafy greens
- garlic
- oily fish

Drink plenty of:

- dandelion tea
- green tea.

What can you do?

In Chinese medicine we look for signs that tell us if anaemia is related to the Liver, the Heart or the Spleen.

Tips for all

- ❀ If you suffer from anaemia during pregnancy, your doctor will prescribe an iron supplement, which may cause constipation (see p. 240).
- ❀ Moxibustion (see p. 333) helps with iron absorption by adding warmth to the body and warming the 'digestive fire'.

❀ Practise moxibustion on St 36 (see p. 112) every day for five minutes. If you feel hot, just do it every other day.

❀ Eat foods from the Blood-nourishing list (see p. 57).

❀ Eat chicken soup (see recipe, p. 314).

❀ Apricots and pumpkin seeds after a meal and foods which are rich in vitamin C all help with the uptake of iron.

And the following should be avoided:

❀ Smoking

❀ Drinking

❀ Coffee

❀ Tea

❀ Antacids

❀ Phosphates in cured meats

Tips by type

Blood Deficiency

Affecting the Liver: Pale, dizzy, blurred vision with floaters, cramps, tingling or numbness in the muscles.

Tongue: Pale, especially the sides (which may also appear slightly orange).

Tips: The Liver type will require rest. Just lying down for thirty minutes in the afternoon will really help.

Affecting the Heart: Pale appearance, especially the lips. Poor concentration and memory, insomnia and anxiety. You may also be experiencing vivid dreams and palpitations.

Tongue: Pale.

Tips: The Heart type will need to pay attention to emotions. How are you feeling about the pregnancy and your circumstances? Is everything in order? Spend time talking through any concerns you might have and give yourself time to focus on becoming a mother and all that means.

Spleen Deficiency (digestive weakness)

Poor appetite and loose stools, gurgling sounds in the abdomen. Exhaustion with a feeling of lifeless and heavy limbs. Breathlessness after the slightest excursion.

Tongue: Pale and swollen.

Tips: The Spleen type will require the most dietary involvement – attention to the rules of eating and protecting the Spleen (see pp. 178–82) should be followed closely.

Hot or Cold

As well as the above, you may well also show signs of either Heat or Cold. If so, follow the basic principles of including heating or warming foods if you feel Cold or cooling foods for Heat (see Food Chart, p. 56).

NETTLES

I know these don't seem like the first choice of delicious things to eat, but nettles are pretty amazing. If we ate more of the simple foods and herbs in our environment, we would not need to take quite so many fancy vitamins and minerals. I do occasionally take supplements, but wherever possible get my nutrients from herbs and foods (and, of course, a good digestion).

Nettles are high in calcium, so if you are not drinking milk or eating dairy, they are a great way to increase your calcium intake. Because of this they help with pain and cramps, both during pregnancy and in the postnatal period.

Nettles are also an excellent source of vitamin K, which is routinely given to the baby at birth. Because of this, nettles help prevent postpartum haemorrhage, making nettle tea the perfect drink leading up to the birth to help increase vitamin K levels.

I have talked to you a great deal about Blood. Well, nettles are a good friend of Blood and blood vessels and therefore are good for preventing varicose veins and haemorrhoids. Furthermore, because nettles are a great Blood tonic and, as we say, 'it takes a drop of mother's blood to make a drop of blood', nettle tea is a great tonic for helping to produce plentiful breast milk.

Nettle Tea

Pick your own fresh nettles. Find a place away from traffic or where dogs might go. Wear rubber or gardening gloves and fill a carrier bag with the tender nettle tops (the top 6–8 leaves of fresh, new plants; if they are in flower, they are too old). When you steep the leaves for tea (a small handful in a pot of boiling water for a few minutes) the stingers will droop and lose their sting.

Nettle Soup

Serves 2
a knob of butter
1 large onion, chopped
2 garlic cloves, chopped
2 large potatoes, finely chopped
1.2 litres (2 pints) fresh nettle leaves (pack gently into a measuring jug)
1.5 litres (2½ pints) chicken or vegetable stock (see p. 254 for chicken
    stock recipe)
fresh chopped parsley
squeeze of lemon juice
nutmeg
freshly ground black pepper

1. Melt the butter, then sauté the onion and garlic. Add the chopped potatoes and toss until the pieces are well coated. Add the nettle leaves and stock, bring to the boil and then lower to a gentle simmer for 20 minutes.
2. Season with chopped parsley, a squeeze of lemon juice, grated nutmeg and plenty of ground black pepper.

Is the Mind on Board?

It's a funny feeling having a secret, especially when that secret is growing inside you. Some of you will want to shout it from the rooftops and others will be more cautious, especially if you had a rocky ride getting pregnant. I remember feeling totally distracted and unable to think of anything else; it was my first thought in the morning and my last before drifting off to sleep. Excitement is a wonderful thing, and it is a great feeling to be able to be excited about something, but you need to try to keep peaceful and calm as well.

It is sometimes hard to know what is a normal response to finding out you are pregnant, and how and when to tell everyone; the truth is, there is probably no such thing as 'normal' here. It's individual and unique, and not something you need worry too much about. My advice is, just don't compare yourself to others, and if you want to tell the world, then do so; equally though, don't feel bad if you want to wait a while.

Anxious feelings

One of the most important jobs I do in my practice is to protect the emotional state of pregnant patients. Many women I see have tried for a long time to conceive and some have lost pregnancies before. Even those who have had a straightforward journey to pregnancy might find themselves bombarded with negativity and fear. I sometimes feel that pregnancy has become all about being worried; it's such a shame.

The tests which are meant to reassure us come with their own level of anxiety; some women are anxious both leading up to and during them, then temporarily reassured, until a new anxiety creeps in. Anxiety reaches epidemic proportions in pregnancy. But although it is vital to be aware of health issues at this time, it is also important to keep a sense of perspective. Every day, all across the world, for thousands of years, women have given birth to healthy babies, safely and without too many difficulties. Of course, problems do occur, but they are the exception and this is helpful to remember.

Irrational feelings, irritability, swinging like a pendulum from bliss to depression, are all considered pretty normal in pregnancy. Some women tell me that because they are feeling physically wretched it's hard to be excited or engaged in their pregnancy, which then leads to feelings of guilt. Others say they are afraid to hope in case it all goes wrong, so they would rather feel pessimistic and be pleasantly surprised. We are complicated creatures and hard to please – no wonder men find us hard to fathom. I usually say that if you are experiencing the full spectrum of emotions, you are probably normal. If the symptoms are prolonged or severe, you may need to speak to your healthcare professional. Sometimes emotional problems can surface during pregnancy and may need addressing professionally. As important as it is to keep things in perspective, it is equally important to know when you require assistance. Sometimes it is when we are at our most vulnerable that we don't seek help, so listen to those you love and trust.

So *how* do we keep things in perspective? It takes a heavy dose of mental strength, and there comes a point when you need to choose what is worth worrying about and what isn't. This practice is called 'cultivation of the mind' in Chinese medicine. There is so much that will happen in your experience as a parent, often wonderful, often completely terrifying. Quite honestly, we owe it to ourselves and our children to choose the things that we allow to keep us awake at night. Don't worry about upsetting people by going *your own way* with things. As my wise mum always says: 'Those that mind don't matter and those that matter don't mind.'

As I have mentioned before, the Heart is the key in terms of balancing your emotions. It is the house of the Shen, which translates as the spirit. To have a good, strong Shen is to be grounded and calm and, yes, serene. Serenity is hard to come by, but something we need to try and hold on to. Just notice how when you are with someone who is serene it automatically has a calming effect on you. Likewise, if you are calm, this will impact on your baby; calm mum = calm baby.

We must be the change we wish to see.
Gandhi

GEORGIE

Georgie was an art teacher at a secondary school. She was pregnant, following IVF, and had to return to work after the summer holiday in the very early stages of pregnancy. She was concerned about the impact of her job on the pregnancy. She said that until she returned to work, she had been sleeping very well and felt rested and calm. As soon as she returned, she found she could not fall asleep easily and was beginning to feel anxious.

I imagine art, and particularly teaching art, is just not one of those things that can been done in a half-hearted way. Up until her return to school Georgie had been very inwardly focused on the pregnancy, but once she was back at school she was on operation output. Teaching takes a lot of Heart, as it is all about communicating, connecting to your students and inspiring – this is the domain of pure Heart energy.

What concerned me was that Georgie would become exhausted, and her tendency then was towards feeling anxious and nervous. In fact, when she arrived for treatment she had a list of concerns. One was that she was 'worried about being stressed'. It's amazing what we find to worry about. It was important to break the cycle.

Together, we went through Georgie's activities and it was clear we needed to build some downtime into her day – some time to retreat, hide even. I suggested that in her lunch hour and breaks she found a place to be alone and lay her head down, or go for a walk in the fresh air. I also recommended that at the end of the day she should go home and lie down on her bed for half an hour. We discussed that television might be too stimulating and to limit computer use in the evenings. Georgie was able to relate to this advice. She said that after her first day back she had gone to watch the telly, then opted for a lie-down on her bed. Sometimes patients just need encouragement that their instincts are actually spot on and worth listening to.

Pregnancy following IVF

Almost all expectant mothers experience some anxiety in the first trimester, but none more so than those who have experienced assisted-pregnancy procedures such as IUI, IVF or egg donation. For these mothers, the journey to conceive successfully has often been long and emotionally and physically gruelling, and the news of a positive pregnancy test can be bittersweet. How do you cope with those nerve-racking first twelve weeks?

Meridian tapping for pregnancy following IVF

It is recommended that all expectant mothers become meridian-tapping experts! Learn the basic points and apply them whenever a fear or anxiety shows up (see p. 35). Tap on whatever you are feeling in the moment until it has reduced to a manageable degree. You can't expect to feel calm all the time and a smidgen of anxiety or awareness is both useful and natural. It is this that will keep you out of the gym or off the alcohol.

The first thing to tap on is believing you are pregnant after all the problems leading to this point, and that the intervention has worked for you:

- ✿ 'Even though I don't believe it, I deeply and completely love and accept myself.'
- ✿ 'Even though I can't be that lucky, I deeply and completely love and accept myself.'
- ✿ 'Even though they have made a mistake, I deeply and completely love and accept myself.'

Many women will have a history of interventions not working, and the fear of disappointment if they allow themselves to believe in their pregnancy and then lose it can be understandably enormous. If this is you, tap as follows:

- ✿ 'Even though it is not safe to believe it, I deeply and completely love and accept myself.'
- ✿ 'Even though I don't dare believe it, I deeply and completely love and accept myself.'
- ✿ 'Even though I am terrified of another disappointment, I deeply and completely love and accept myself.'

❀ 'Even though I can't allow myself to hope, I deeply and completely love and accept myself.'

Visualize your embryo growing every day. Imagine sending love to it and supporting it as it develops. Connect with it. Visualize a strong attachment to the lining of your womb.

While twinges and aches and pains are normal as your body adjusts to pregnancy, they can seem terrifying. If this happens to you, tap on your thoughts and feelings, but also the physical symptoms themselves:

❀ 'Even though I have this ache on the right side of my abdomen, I deeply and completely love and accept myself.'
❀ 'Even though I get these twinges, I deeply and completely love and accept myself.'

The chances are that you will be able to reduce the symptoms that way, and, in doing so, will also calm yourself down.

Emotions and the organs

It is quite normal in a well-balanced life to experience the whole spectrum of emotions. However, it is when we become stuck in one, or when it becomes overwhelming so that it impacts on the rest of our life that it needs our attention. Emotions we might have repressed for many years may come to the surface during pregnancy and require our attention. It is all part of the process.

In Chinese medicine, the organs are associated with different emotions:

❀ **Liver** Frustration, anger and our drive in life
❀ **Heart** Joy, excitement, but can suffer with anxiety
❀ **Spleen** Pensiveness, worry and ability to nurture both ourselves and others
❀ **Lungs** Grief, sadness and our connection to the world
❀ **Kidneys** Fear, fright and our willpower

Anxiety
Tips by type
Blood Deficiency

Blood Deficiency can easily affect the Heart, leading to poor memory and anxiety with palpitations. There can be difficulty falling asleep and you might feel easily startled.

Tongue: Pale, orange-tinged at the sides.

Tips: Rest is important. Increase Blood-nourishing foods (see p. 57). Acupressure: P 6 (see p. 109).

Yin Deficiency

This is similar in that it can affect the Heart, leading to anxiety, but in this picture there is more restlessness and feelings of heat. Generally, you will feel a bit irritable and overstimulated. You are your own worst enemy, as you don't know how to stop and say 'No', but you need time out.

I sometimes see this pattern in women who had a difficult path to pregnancy, and who may have done fertility treatment. They often enter pregnancy 'on empty' and carry on with life, work and love with the same 100 per cent commitment they always did. If this applies, you might need to rethink, slow down, say 'No' more and prioritize yourself and the baby. Learning to relax now will serve you well over the first year of motherhood.

Tongue: Peeled; looks as if area of coating scraped away.

Tips: Say no to a few things, instead of filling every waking hour with work. Value downtime and make it a priority. Just be. Learn to meditate. This is a gift of life and will serve you well. Acupressure: P 6 (see p. 109).

Fire

When there is too much heat build-up in the body over a period of time, it turns into what's known in Chinese medicine as 'fire'. This makes you feel very agitated and restless, with powerful emotional symptoms, such as outbursts of anger. There is often a strong thirst and there can be a bitter or scorched taste in the mouth. A practitioner can often identify fire through smell.

There may be a history of alcohol use or recreational drugs, but these are by no means the only causes of fire. Women who have had many IVF cycles often present with too much fire, especially in the Liver (see also Yin Deficiency, above).

On an emotional level your mood may be extreme at times and you may need to seek professional help to deal with anger or deep-seated mind issues.

Tongue: Red body with yellow coating.

Tips: • Avoid all heating foods and substances (see p. 58).
- Heavy fatty foods and chocolate are not good for fire as they are heavy to digest and can make the problem worse.
- You need to cool down on every level, so start replacing any heating substance like chocolate, coffee and alcohol (hopefully you are not still drinking these anyway) with cooling drinks and foods, like mint or chamomile tea, and lots of fruits and vegetables.
- Walk away from conflict and try to be around people who make you feel calm.
- Don't over exercise, especially in hot environments.
- Try to let off steam with a gentle stroll in a green space.

Stagnation

This type of anxiety is less intense, but still you might be feeling low in mood, frustrated, mildly irritable with an underlying feeling of depression. You may feel emotionally stuck or stagnant in your personal situation, frustrated about your life or angry with someone. And you might sigh a lot and feel generally fed up!

Tongue: Mauve.

Tips: Make sure you are getting enough movement throughout your body and you are not stuck sitting behind a computer all day. It is good to have direction and focus, and you may feel this is lacking. Formulating some sort of plan – if you draw out what your needs and your desires are – will help you to clarify things and ease your frustrations. Acupressure: Liv 3 (see p. 112).

Patients with the Blood-Deficient and Yin-Deficient patterns usually affecting the Heart will benefit from introducing rituals into their week (see p. 187). Try to set time aside for yoga and meditation and anything that encourages you to switch off and relax. Repetitive, non-talking activities are best, sewing, yoga or any hobby that requires little output in energy. You are less likely to benefit from talking therapies although you might feel drawn to them as you usually enjoy 'doing'. My advice is practise 'being' instead. You need to learn to step out of life occasionally and to retreat inwards; look for peace within yourself.

FEAR AND THE KIDNEYS

Fear is the emotion connected to the Kidneys and, in some women, it is an ever-present emotion. It takes on two forms: one being a chronic state of anxiety, the other a sudden, acute fright. The sudden-fright variety is said to make the Kidney Qi descend, and since the Kidney and the Bladder are partners, you can see this relationship demonstrated in wetting one's knickers following a fright! The chronic-anxiety type is more common in pregnancy.

I see many women enter pregnancy with poor Kidney energy. Years of working long hours, fear surrounding their ability to conceive, being an older first-time mother, repeated IVF treatments (which can be emotionally and physically draining) and the general fear culture in which we exist – all of these things impact on Kidney energy and, ultimately, make you feel more anxious and more fearful.

The problem with starting pregnancy with poor Kidney function is that pregnancy itself drains the Kidneys, so it becomes harder to correct the imbalance, unless you are committed to resting and you really learn to face your fears. Otherwise, it becomes a bit of a vicious cycle, in which fear and anxiety grow as the Kidney energy depletes.

I don't want to go on too much about this, as there is enough pressure on women as it is. But we all need to learn to rest and preserve our energies better. Some of us have become compulsive 'do-ers', by which I mean we are always on the go and understand little about rest and relaxation. We work hard all week and then, at the end of the day, when we are exhausted, we go and work out, draining what little energy we have left out of our bones – literally (remember the connection between the Kidneys and the bones – see p. 19). Yoga is on the increase, but this is sometimes taught by people who understand little about energy. Working out in an overheated room when you are trying to conceive, are pregnant or have just had a baby is a really bad idea. You might feel better temporarily because the vigorous activity moves stagnant Qi. The question is, how do you feel in the morning? Or generally throughout the day? That temporary boost of energy is like the buzz from a coffee or a shot of wheat grass; these are quick-fix solutions, but they do not last and they deplete your energy.

Like everything in Chinese medicine, I need to add here that it does, to a large extent, depend on the individual. Of course, some of you out there, the ones with big ear lobes (a sign of good, strong Kidneys) and strong bones and back – you can run and run without so much as an ache in your bones. So this section is not for you. But for the rest of us mere mortals, it's a good idea to preserve the Kidney energy, as you never know when you might need the strength and adrenalin to run away from a tiger (or, more likely, stay up late at night nursing your newborn baby).

Yoga for anxiety
Yoga tip: be here now, stay in the present moment.
Practice: humming breath (*bhramari*)
Worry is the work of pregnancy and many women experience intense anxiety at least some of the time during their pregnancy. Yoga breath and mindfulness are highly effective tools to prevent and relieve anxiety.[16] The main reason it works so well is because when we focus on each and every breath it keeps us fully grounded in the present moment, and taking things one breath at a time is a manageable way to handle any challenge.

You can do this practice sitting up or lying down, whichever is most comfortable:

Close your eyes and let your breath flow freely and easily, perhaps following the instructions for the full yogic breath (see p. 196 – the remedy for exhaustion). Have your lips gently closed. After a few breaths, allow your focus to rest mostly with the exhale. Let the inhale take care of itself. When you next exhale, hum softly as the breath leaves. Let the hum continue until the end of the breath. Continue like this, humming as every breath leaves. The sound does not need to be very loud or very long. Just enough for you and your baby to feel the gentle vibrations of the humming sound deep in your body. You can direct the sound down to your heart. You can cover your ears with your hands to take your attention deeper within, as you listen to the hum. The most important thing is to keep the eyes closed and your mind fully focused on the sound and feel of the hum.

This practice will calm you, and the sonic massage will also soothe your baby. It works like magic. Every time. (For more yoga breathing and sound practices, listen to *Mother's Breath* – see Resources, p. 343; and for more information on Uma Dinsmore-Tuli's books and websites, and yoga in pregnancy, please see Resources, p. 339, and Further Reading, p. 347.)

Miscarriage

Sadly, I have seen many women through miscarriage, and I myself had two. Although it's still not something that people talk about much, women are more open than they once were, when these things were only whispered about, and you would be amazed at how many people are willing to share their stories by way of support when the subject is broached.

I do not believe acupuncture, or any treatment for that matter, can save a pregnancy that is not viable. However, there are times when some early support might help a pregnancy along. I have treated women with threatened miscarriage when early intervention has been able to direct a fragile pregnancy in 'the right direction'. Of course, there is no way of knowing if these pregnancies would have survived anyway. But the point is that some do.

Miscarriage is often not taken particularly seriously in Western medicine, unless it results in complications. Many women go straight back into work, sometimes the following day. Chinese medicine takes a different view and considers the experience to be as draining as childbirth. There is also the emotional impact of miscarriage to consider, particularly when the pregnancy has taken a long time to conceive or was a result of IVF.

Why do miscarriages occur?

About half of all fertilized embryos never implant or do not implant well enough to become a pregnancy. Sometimes, a woman may sense she was briefly pregnant, or may even get a faint early positive pregnancy test, but then it fails to progress.

Most miscarriages occur in the first trimester, and approximately 15 per cent of all pregnancies will end in miscarriage.

The reasons for miscarriage are not easy to establish. Possible causes include the idea that the woman's body is rejecting a problem with a pregnancy; that there are hormonal imbalances; problems with the sperm, uterus, implantation, placenta, cervix or immune system; or that an infection has caused the miscarriage.

Miscarriage terminology

When a miscarriage happens in the first twelve weeks, it is referred to as an early miscarriage; between twelve and twenty-four weeks, it is defined as a late miscarriage; after this time, the age of foetal viability, the term stillbirth (see p. 151) is used.

Threatened miscarriage

This is where a woman might experience warning signs of a miscarriage, including bleeding, lower-back ache and abdominal cramps. The cervix is still closed, though, and there will be evidence from an ultrasound that the foetus is still viable.

Inevitable miscarriage

This is where miscarriage is already happening or is about to, and can't be prevented, signalled by the cervix beginning to dilate.

Missed miscarriage

This is where it is discovered that the foetus no longer has a heartbeat, usually during a routine scan. There are often no warning signs, although many women realize once they notice that their morning sickness has suddenly stopped. Depending on the individual circumstances, it might be left for a couple of weeks to see if the miscarriage will occur naturally. In early pregnancy, a small operation similar to a dilation and curettage, called an ERPC (evacuation of retained products of conception), might be performed, where the foetus is surgically removed; or medical treatment may be given to hasten the onset of miscarriage.

Ectopic pregnancy

An ectopic pregnancy is when the fertilized egg implants outside the womb. This usually occurs in a Fallopian tube or, less commonly, can occur in an ovary, the cervix or abdominal space. The pregnancy can't be saved, but early diagnosis and treatment improve the chances of being able to have a normal pregnancy at a later date.

Note: Always tell your midwife or GP if you have bleeding. Signs of miscarriage usually include: pain, heavy bleeding with clots and sometimes a dragging-down sensation.

After a miscarriage

Following a miscarriage, it's essential to establish that it is complete, as there is a possibility that not all placental products will have been discharged. In this case, an ERPC may be needed to make sure the uterus is free of all the tissue that needs to come out. This small operation is performed under general anaesthetic.

Most of the work I do around miscarriage is helping women to recover, and also helping women who have had miscarriages in the past with support through their subsequent pregnancies.

Qi and Blood are important considerations following a miscarriage, particularly if there has been heavy blood loss. Following the guidelines for nourishing Qi and Blood (see pp. 26 and 33) and taking adequate time to recover are all-important here. The recipes and store cupboard in the post-natal section of this book will also help you with food choices. Raspberry-leaf tea is an excellent tonic, as is nettle tea. Aubergines help move Blood, and have a strong tonifying effect on the uterus.

I also think that herbal medicine has an important role to play in miscarriage recovery, but this is a highly specialized area and beyond the scope of this book. I would urge you, however, to see a qualified herbalist (see Resources, p. 339).

In terms of the emotions, my experience is that some women will want to 'get back to normal' as quickly as possible. For many, this approach works just fine and they are happier getting on with their lives, rather than wanting to dwell on their sadness and the loss. If this is you, that's fine, but just be sure it is really how you are feeling and that you are not just acting that way for everyone else's sake. Other women will find it much harder to recover and I have met some who are haunted by the loss for many years.

Men too suffer during a miscarriage, as they also experience the emotions of loss. Clearly, they are not going through the physical process of losing a longed-for baby, but emotionally it can be hard for them to know how to help. It's difficult when your partner is sad and inconsolable, but there is no need to suffer in silence.

Here are some useful suggestions to help you through:

❀ Give yourself some emotional and physical time out – your body is pumped full of pregnancy hormones and the drop in these will contribute to feelings of sadness. Your breasts may have grown and your abdomen may have swollen, which will make you feel as if you are still pregnant, possibly adding to your sadness.

❀ Take time to grieve. This is a very important part of the recovery process.

❀ Try to take your mind off what has happened, but rather than do this by throwing yourself into work, try to do it through pleasurable things.

❀ Don't expect too much of yourself.

Stillbirth

Stillbirth occurs in fewer than 1 per cent of pregnancies and is where the baby dies in the womb before birth. The term stillbirth applies if this happens from twenty-four weeks on. For some women, this means that labour has to be induced, and in some cases the baby dies during labour. I must emphasize how rare this is because it is naturally a fear experienced by many women during pregnancy.

Why does it happen?

It's not always possible to answer this question. It may be that the baby could not thrive or develop normally. In some cases, it is because the placenta has deteriorated and the baby hasn't been able to get enough oxygen. The liver condition that can occur in pregnancy, obstetric cholestasis, can result in still-birth, which is why it is so important to monitor this condition closely. And premature delivery can cause too much stress to a small and vulnerable baby.

Tapping exercise following miscarriage (from Emma Roberts)
A miscarriage, however early on, requires a grieving process: grieving for the lost baby, grieving for the lost dreams and hopes. Take some time for yourself, allow the sorrow to come to the surface and gently tap as you sit with it (see

p. 35). This will help to take some of the intensity away, but it will not entirely clear the sadness until your unconscious mind deems it safe to release it. It is a natural process which tapping can support, but which is healthy to go through.

Miscarriage brings up many conflicting thoughts and emotions, especially when it is unexplained. Women are often told it is 'just one of those things' – that 'it happens to many women'. This may be true, but it does not address the emotional impact of the loss. Miscarriage is usually nature's way of releasing an unviable pregnancy, and no one is to blame – however, many women become racked with guilt, thinking that it is somehow their fault, if only they hadn't done this or that. If you are feeling similar guilt, tap as follows:

- ❀ 'Even though it is all my fault, I deeply and completely love and accept myself.'
- ❀ 'Even though I must have done something wrong, I deeply and completely love and accept myself.'
- ❀ 'Even though I should/shouldn't have done X, I deeply and completely love and accept myself.'
- ❀ 'Even though my body failed me, I deeply and completely love and accept myself.'

Other useful tapping phrases are as follows:

- ❀ 'Even though I have this miscarriage shock, I deeply and completely love and accept myself.'
- ❀ 'Even though I have these miscarriage emotions, I deeply and completely love and accept myself.'
- ❀ 'Even though I have this miscarriage trauma, I deeply and completely love and accept myself.'

Once you have had time to release the most highly charged emotions, tell yourself, or a therapist, the story of what happened, stopping to tap on any piece of it that has emotional intensity attached. For example, maybe you had spotting, in which case you would use words such as:

'Even though I have this spotting emotion, I deeply and completely love and accept myself.'

It is impossible to put into words the grief associated with losing a newborn baby. It is one of life's greatest injustices, and I have sadly treated a few women over the years following the loss of their babies. Simply being a kind and listening source of support for these women can help them through this time. (See Resources, p. 339, for more information on support services.)

When to start trying again

The temptation is sometimes to try for another baby as soon as possible to replace the loss. That can work out well for some couples; it really depends on the nature of the miscarriage. My first miscarriage was very early, at seven weeks, and I conceived my second daughter the following month. However, my second miscarriage was much later, and I was quite unwell, having suffered from significant blood loss which meant I had to stay in hospital for several days. After that, I made the decision not to put myself through it again. My view was that I had two daughters and I was already blessed. It's very individual, and no one can say what the right response is. Had I decided to have another go after the second miscarriage, I think I would have needed a full four months to get over it physically (maybe longer emotionally). Of course, age is a consideration but even so, it is usually better to enter a subsequent pregnancy in good health than to rush into it too soon.

My approach

My recommendations for patients who have miscarried will vary according to the circumstances and the person:

- ❀ If there is a history of miscarriage, I will spend time correcting any energetic imbalances and my advice will follow the pre-conception plan in this book. (A more detailed plan can be found in my previous book, *The Baby-Making Bible*.)
- ❀ In the case of a threatened miscarriage, I will try to see if we can apply some treatment to save the pregnancy. Acupuncture will not save a pregnancy with a genetic abnormality, but in many other cases there may be some hope.
- ❀ After a miscarriage, it's important to regain your balance in terms of your health before trying again. I address this with each patient.

chapter ten
SECOND TRIMESTER (WEEKS 13–27)

In the second trimester, many women begin to notice that the discomfort of nausea, along with the initial anxieties related to being pregnant, eases, and a sense of confidence and bloom develops. There is a lovely phrase in Chinese medicine – 'making the prosperity blossom'. And that's just what you can do more of during the second trimester through your lifestyle, diet and your emotions, as you start to get more used to the idea of being pregnant, begin to tell friends and colleagues and build your energy in preparation for the third trimester, birth and the first few steps of motherhood.

Is the Engine Working?

For your baby, the second trimester is a time of rapid growth and organ development. For you, your energy is likely to return and this is the perfect time to catch up on healthy eating and also relaxing into your pregnancy.

How your baby develops

During the second trimester, your baby's skeleton and organs mature. Growth is rapid – in the fourteenth and fifteenth weeks alone your baby will put on half its own bodyweight twice in two weeks. Fingers and toes become more defined and the bones and muscles continue to develop. Your baby's face changes by the day and by week 15 hair has begun to grow: head hair, eyelashes, eyebrows and fine hairs all over the body.

By week 16, your baby's fingerprints are set and the lips are much more defined. By this time, your baby can use its fast-growing muscles to curl its toes and make a fist. In week 17, fat stores begin to be laid down – another key factor for growth.

In week 18, when you are likely to have an ultrasound, the foetus will have reached the end of the first big growth phase, measuring around 13.5cm and weighing about 150g. The brain is already active, triggering the heart-beat, digestion and movement. External noises can be detected, so if a loud bang makes you jump your baby might jump too.

The kidneys begin to function and pass a small amount of urine and, by week 19, your baby can hear. A scan at this stage in your pregnancy will give you the opportunity to find out if you are having a boy or a girl, if you want to know. In a first pregnancy, you will probably feel your baby move around week 20, usually earlier in later pregnancies. The first flutter or movement might be just that, a 'quickening'.

Your metabolic rate increases, making you energized and also more hungry. Progesterone relaxes your muscles and ligaments in preparation for delivery, so you might feel more supple and flexible than usual. Take care of your body though, as it is easy to damage slackened ligaments. Progesterone also has sedative effects, which may mean you start to feel more relaxed and confident. You might also get a dose of 'baby brain', as the relaxing effects of progesterone can make you a bit forgetful and you may find that you can't seem to concentrate on anything.

By the end of this second trimester, your baby has a chance of surviving if born, although intensive care would be needed.

CHINESE MEDICINE AND THE SECOND TRIMESTER

In Chinese medicine, the second trimester is all about creating a healthy balance, both for you and your baby. Advice centres around avoiding foods that are either too Cold or too Hot (see p. 177 for nutrition in the second trimester), nourishing the Spleen, which is your engine when it comes to digestion, eating little and often and keeping a calm outlook. You're probably just beginning to get your appetite back, so this is the perfect time to think a bit more about engaging with nutritious food again, if it's been a struggle up to now. Good eating habits at this time will help you make good Blood, which in turn is nourishing for your baby. But don't be tempted to overeat as your appetite returns, as indigestion and heartburn, too much 'stomach fire', can become more common during the second trimester.

The general advice for exercise is summed up, as with food, by 'not too little, not too much' and listen to your own body to become aware of what is right for you as an individual. If you are working at a desk all day, then don't sit for too long periods at a time – get up and move around every hour or so to keep your Qi moving. As I know from personal experience, Stagnation can be an issue in the second trimester, which we see in the common conditions like oedema. Chinese medicine talks of 'moving the four limbs' to keep the Qi flowing well, and the best way to do this is by going for walks. Likewise, when it comes to rest try to get a good night's sleep (see p. 193 for advice on insomnia), but don't be tempted to sleep in too much or you may become a little sluggish.

Your energy reserves will start to replenish through the second trimester with any luck and, alongside a renewed sense of energy, you might be feeling more sociable and less exhausted, so do enjoy yourself while keeping mindful of your body.

A WORD TO PARTNERS

Pregnancy offers a window of time to adjust to your new role. Even before your baby arrives, your partner's needs are changing and it's an opportunity for you to change too. Think about beginning to shift some of your less healthy habits. If you still smoke, consider giving up or, at the very least, smoke outside the house. Cut down on nights out and alcohol too. There is no need to become a saint, but small adjustments on your part will help your partner with the huge ones she is making.

Help your partner with chores that maybe you did not do before. And if she goes to bed earlier than normal, perhaps lie on the bed with her for ten minutes before she sleeps, and spend that time stroking her growing bump and having a little chat to your baby growing inside. It may seem daft, but the baby will hear your voice.

The film *March of the Penguins*, which explores the breeding cycles of the emperor penguins, shows how the young penguin can recognize the sound of its father's voice in a crowd of literally thousands of other penguins, and so find its way back to him. This can make it easier to understand how your baby might also recognize your voice and find it a comfort once born. But don't worry if this does not come naturally to you; there are many different kinds of fathers and you will find your own way.

Antenatal Check-ups and Tests

Depending on where you live, you are likely to have ten antenatal check-ups for your first pregnancy, if there are no complications that need closer monitoring or treatment. After your initial booking appointment (see p. 97), these visits should take place at weeks 16, 25, 28, 31, 34, 36, 38, 40 and 41 (if you haven't already had your baby by then). For subsequent pregnancies, you will probably have seven antenatal visits at weeks 16, 28, 34, 36, 38 and 41.

You will be offered an ultrasound at around weeks 18–20 (the 'Anomaly Scan') to check your baby's development and the position of your placenta. From around twenty-four weeks, your midwife will start measuring the size of your bump to get an idea of how your baby is growing, and from thirty-six weeks, she may 'palpate' (feel) your bump to check what position your baby is in. If there are any concerns you may be referred for an ultrasound.

Diagnostic tests

If screening tests indicate that your baby has a high risk of Down's syndrome, you will be offered a diagnostic test which can tell for certain. You should also be offered counselling at this point, so do ask for it if you are not. The tests include a more detailed ultrasound scan, amniocentesis to test the amniotic fluid and chorionic villus sampling (CVS) to check placental cells. Amniocentesis and CVS are invasive, involving the insertion of needles, and do carry their own risks. All of which means it is crucial to talk through the risks and benefits of any tests during pregnancy as they are ultimately your choice.

Where to Have Your Baby

A midwife's role throughout your pregnancy is one of advocacy, even if you are not fortunate enough to be cared for by the same midwife for the whole journey. It's good to start thinking about your options for where to have your baby early; and don't be afraid to change your mind or be flexible as your pregnancy develops.

Depending on where you live and your personal health circumstances, your health team will chat through with you the pros and cons of the various options available to you. For example, if you live in a city you might feel very comfortable with the thought of a home birth, knowing that the hospital is only minutes away, if needed. If you live in a more rural location, the time it would take to get to hospital in the event of any, albeit unlikely, complications will be a factor you'll consider with the midwife.

Do ask around for differing opinions if you're not 100 per cent convinced by what you hear; I know many women who only discovered home birth was an option after they had had their baby and hadn't thought to even ask about it. The other major factor is listening to your own instincts. For some women, the thought of giving birth at home is incredibly empowering and comforting. They feel they will be relaxed, be able to make their own food, potter around and have all their favourite things within arm's reach. But for other women, the thoughts of 'what might go wrong' are too overwhelming and would cancel out all the potential benefits of being at home. Go with whatever gives you confidence and makes you feel comfortable.

Hospital

Some hospitals now have midwifery-led units. If you are going to give birth in one of these units you will meet the full team and these same people will be there for the big day. They are often located on the same level as the hospital birth unit, where you would be transferred if there were any complications. Midwifery units can almost feel like home from home, as the number-one aim is to achieve as natural a birth as possible.

If your hospital doesn't have a midwifery-led unit, you will be given a tour of the birth unit. Unfortunately, you will be unlikely to meet the midwife who will be present for the birth, but you can still get a good feel for the place, and the majority of hospitals now try to create as homely an atmosphere as possible. The main thing is to know what it will be like ahead of time and feel prepared, rather than be in for any surprises.

Home

Very few women in the UK give birth at home – only around 2.5 per cent – even though women who do so tend to labour well at home with good outcomes, less intervention and good recovery. In the Netherlands, as many as a third of women have home births, with outcomes as good as hospital births. Any woman can request a home birth, so if it's not offered as an option, you should always feel you can ask to talk it through. Even if you decide to go with the hospital option, just knowing there are choices is definitely worthwhile.

It's essential that you get to know and trust your midwife over time, if you are keen to consider a home birth. That way you feel safe and cared for and, therefore, more confident and relaxed through the birth. You will have two midwives during labour, the second being called in once birth is imminent.

You do need to be well prepared for coping with labour if you decide that a home birth is the best option.

Whatever your decision, I have included a whole chapter on preparing for labour (see pp. 246–59), which in itself is a great grounding for becoming a mum.

TRUDY – ON BEING AN OLDER MUM

When people realize I had a first child aged forty, I am often asked: Didn't you hear your biological clock ticking? The honest answer is, 'No.' To complete the metaphor, I was probably telling the time with a DIY sundial using the shadows of the trees. Aged thirty-nine, I was completely oblivious to age-related hormone profiles, infertility issues and such like. In my blissfully ignorant Peter Pan state, I was having the time of my life. I had a fantastic job, dining out as and when, and travelling the world.

After suffering postpartum thyroiditis and a run of miscarriages, several years later, in the clear light of day, I realize how exceptional it was to fall pregnant in just six months. I still pinch myself to confirm how lucky I was to give birth to a healthy son.

When I think about what I've been through these last years, physically and emotionally, I tell myself that all these things – good and bad – could have happened in my twenties or thirties. What I didn't realize though, was that health issues relating to conception and pregnancy take longer to diagnose, resolve and bypass, than one imagines. Diagnosis for my thyroid problems took eighteen months alone.

With the benefit of hindsight, would I do it differently? Probably not. But I would ensure any daughter of mine was properly briefed. Women have come a long way in terms of having choices. My dear grandmother never had the vote, let alone the chance of a fulfilling career. Two generations later, we need prompting to continue to excel in our careers and our personal lives, and the courage to make active choices.

I wish a wise fairy godmother had whispered in my ear when I was twenty-nine: 'You've honed your CV, honey; now, in the same way, it's time to visualize a life plan, for you, a partner and children. Yes, my dear, you can have it all. Remember, thanks to other women before us, mothers are now the most protected species in the workplace.'

Multiples (Twins or More)

A multiple pregnancy makes greater demands on the body, so being fit and healthy before you even conceive can be a real bonus here, as can eating well and generally taking good care of yourself during your pregnancy.

Some of the common conditions that women experience in pregnancy can be amplified for women having twins, including pregnancy nausea (see p. 107), tiredness (see p. 115) and anaemia (see p. 134). The advice to get all the rest you need is therefore even more important if you are having twins, and ensure that you are getting plenty of iron-rich foods in your diet (see p. 130). High blood pressure (see p. 221) and fluid-retention-related conditions (see pp. 211–220) are also more common for twin pregnancies, so it's a good idea to read up on these sections ahead of time to help prevent them, rather than have to tackle them head-on once symptoms have set in.

OSTEOPATHY AND PREGNANCY

During pregnancy, your body needs to adapt to carrying your growing baby, changing your relationship to gravity. Osteopathy will identify stresses and strains related to your history and recognize postural compensations.

How is your posture?

Where do you carry your weight when standing, which part of your foot – ankle, arch or toes? Clinically, I find most people to be posterior, with all their weight going through their heels and ankles. Eighty per cent of your body weight should be balanced by the arch of your foot, to enable your body to deal with the day-to-day forces of being up against gravity, to translate the various surfaces upon which you walk and to enable the body to do this effectively and efficiently. You can put a sticker on your mobile phone to remind yourself to remain aware, and to correct as necessary by softening your knees.

How do you breathe?

Not many people are aware of the way in which posture relates to breathing and, in turn, blood flow. When you slouch with round shoulders and scrunch up your body, you disturb the efficiency of blood flow, which can make it stagnant and suboptimal, thereby affecting your health.

The aim of breathing deeply is to send a regular and plentiful supply of fresh oxygenated blood around the body, so as to deliver the nutrients needed to repair and grow and to remove toxins from your system. Breathing from your diaphragm also helps you to remain connected to yourself, so that you do not get lost in the detail of the outside world.

How do you sit? Does your work/home environment support well-being?

The way in which you organize your space, such as your driving seat and your desk, are key in helping you to keep correct posture. This is especially important if you have a desk job or spend a lot of time at the wheel of your car.

Set up your workstation with your screen at eye level. Keep your shoulders, elbows and wrists in alignment and supported when you are working. This will balance mechanical stresses and help maintain optimum breathing and hence blood supply.

How does your body react in times of stress and other strong emotional states?

The best thing you can do in terms of managing your body alignment is to become aware of how your body reacts to life events, such as times of stress – be they physical or emotional. For example, you may hunch your shoulders when you are tense, or you may find that you clench your fists or your jaw – putting strain on your arms and shoulders or head. By raising your awareness of how you tend to react, you can learn how to deal with stress in healthier ways.

What position do you sleep in?

You spend about a third of your life asleep, so it's vital that you make sure your sleeping position is safe. When you sleep, make sure your body is in an optimum position to help the spine align, ensuring a good supply of blood to all of your body. This means your spine being in a straight line. You will need someone else to check this for you at some stage, as it's hard to tell by yourself if your spine is in a straight line. It may mean having two pillows under your head and one between your knees and ankles while you sleep on your side.

Sleeping is a very individual activity, so it's impossible to say that one particular type of mattress is right for everybody. The key thing is to make sure you are keeping a correct sleeping posture, as described above – and that you find your bed comfortable and an inviting place to be.

The above information has been kindly provided by Maxine Hamilton Stubber.

Common Conditions

Nosebleeds

Nosebleeds are a nuisance, but it is normal to experience them more often during pregnancy, especially from the second trimester onwards.

Why do they happen?

Pregnancy hormones make your blood vessels dilate and your increased blood supply at this time puts more pressure on your veins, sometimes causing them to break open and bleed. A sudden nosebleed where the blood is bright red can be a sign of too much Heat in the body.

What can you do?

Consider if you are generating too much Heat through stress or diet. Once you've had a nosebleed, the following can also help:

- ❄ Apply some ice on the bridge of the nose.
- ❄ Pinch the tip of your nose for five to ten minutes.
- ❄ Lean forward rather than back to drain the blood through your nose, rather than down your throat.
- ❄ An elastic band around the knuckles of the fingers.

Lower-back pain/pelvic-girdle pain

Many women experience pain in the joints during pregnancy, and many more experience discomfort in the lower back; this is the part of the body that is most stressed by the additional weight you are carrying.

Why does it happen?

Pregnancy hormones relax your joints, ligaments and muscles, which also creates added stress on these areas, causing pain.

What can you do?

Often, pain can be treated quickly with one acupuncture treatment. I also find the combination of acupuncture and osteopathy to be very effective.[17]

Reflexology too can be very helpful in relieving tension and pain in the spinal area (thoracic and lumbar) by strengthening the muscles and increasing the circulation and nerve impulses.

Reflex areas to treat
Starting at the base of your thumb, take twelve steps (representing the twelve upper vertebrae) using the 'caterpillar' technique (see p. 335) along the bone to the edge of the wrist. Continue around the bone for five further steps (middle-lower vertebrae) until you hit the middle of the wrist which is the coccyx – hold this point and make circles for ten seconds. Repeat three times.

Reflexology for pelvic-girdle pain
Simply rotate your ankles both clockwise and anti-clockwise for several minutes every day. In reflexology terms the ankle area corresponds with the hips, so by making your ankles more flexible, your pelvic area will benefit too.

If you are suffering badly, I would recommend visiting a reflexologist, who can apply a variety of techniques to help ease the aches and pains, alongside balancing your emotions (too complicated to work yourself!).

Yoga for pelvic-girdle pain
Yoga tip: keep weight evenly balanced, and use muscles to support the pelvis.
Practice: the pelvic scoop
Yoga postures and mindful movements can ease pain in the lower back and the pelvic girdle.

The single most useful point to bear in mind if you are experiencing pain in the pelvic joints is to keep your weight evenly balanced through both feet and legs. Standing, sitting, getting in and out of cars, always consider how to move the weight down through both legs: take smaller steps, avoid standing on one leg, keep both feet on the ground when you sit down, and when you get into a car, turn sideways and do it bum first, then swing both legs around together. Do the same when you get out, turning in the seat and getting both feet down before you stand. These commonsense everyday changes make a huge difference to pain levels.

The second most helpful yoga tool to ease pelvic and lower-back pain is to use your muscles consciously to create support for your pelvis. Squeeze the buttocks when you rise to your feet and when you walk: the buttock muscles are strong enough to provide a lot of support for your pelvis. Also, contract the pelvic-floor muscles to provide support from beneath, and squeeze in the lowest and deepest layer of abdominal muscle to support the pubic bones.

> The best way to do this effectively is to stand with your feet hip-width apart and knees bent. Keep the arches of the feet well lifted – they support your lower back. Then imagine that you have a long tail attached to your coccyx and as you inhale, stick out your imaginary tail behind you, reaching it towards the bottom of the wall behind you, lengthening and deepening the curve in your lower back. As you breathe out, let the imaginary tail descend, and then tuck it right underneath you, like a dog putting its tail between its legs. Squeeze your buttocks as you tuck the tail through. Let this movement scoop your pelvis forwards, rounding off the curve in your lower back. Straighten your knees as you carry this movement forward, and feel the contraction in the belly muscles underneath your bump, just above your pubic bones. Repeat at least a dozen times or more: knees bent, tail back and down, then squeeze the buttocks, move the tail under and through, lift and scoop as you straighten your knees. Link each scoop into the next, like a series of little circles. Allow the scooping movement of your pelvis to move upwards through the spine until the whole spine and neck undulates.

For more information on Uma Dinsmore-Tuli's books and website, and yoga in pregnancy, please see Resources, p. 339, and Further Readings, p. 347.

CANDIDA

Candida has been a bit of a hot topic for some years now, and I see lots of women who have been put on very restrictive diets in order to help eradicate an overgrowth of Candida.

Candida is a yeast that normally occurs in the gut, but, in certain circumstances, it is given the opportunity to grow out of control. Pregnancy is one of these times, and also certain medications seem to lead to its growth, such as steroids and antibiotics. Diet too plays a role and an overgrowth of Candida may indicate that the woman is low in iron, or is developing gestational diabetes (see p. 172).

Candida is not a threat to either mother or baby, but it can be stubborn and can cause breastfeeding problems later. This is because it can be passed from the mother's breast to the baby's mouth. Most nutritionists advise not treating Candida during pregnancy, but you can keep it at bay by cleaning up your diet, having your iron levels checked and following the recommendations for Damp (see p. 31).

Haemorrhoids or piles/varicose veins and vulval varicosities

During pregnancy, the veins are under increased pressure to perform their job of circulating the blood around the body. The blood may collect in the veins so that they become congested, distended and protruding; the common sites for this problem are the rectum, the vulva and the lower legs.

Haemorrhoids or piles are the grape-like veins that protrude from the rectum. They often start quite small, but can grow quite easily, starting as mild distension with a little fresh blood and progressing to cause more swelling, itching and sometimes pain. As with most pregnancy ailments, it is best to catch and treat early if possible. (For treatment, see tips below.)

Vulval varicosities are veins that protrude around the vulva or vagina; these veins do not bleed, but can cause pain and itching. (For treatment, see tips below.)

Thrombophlebitis is a clot in the superficial vein of the legs, causing reddening and tenderness. The treatment for this is rest and elevation (of the leg) and a support stocking.

Note: A complication of these conditions is that they can develop into deep-vein thrombosis (DVT) – a clot in the vein in the calf. The legs will feel painful and heavy. You must see your midwife or GP as this can at worst develop into a pulmonary embolism. Treatment for this is rest, elevation and support stockings, as well as injections to thin the blood (anticoagulants).

Tips for all

- ✿ Epsom-salt baths: pour four cups of Epsom salts into your bath water. Soak for twenty minutes, then lie down and rest for fifteen minutes after your bath.
- ✿ Apply witch hazel or lemon juice locally. Witch hazel herb can also be used – dilute 115g of the dried herb in boiling water and leave to seep overnight or for eight hours; add this to a shallow basin you can put in the bath to sit in and bathe the haemorrhoids.
- ✿ Wear support stockings.
- ✿ Avoid clothing that restricts the blood flow and avoid sitting cross-legged.
- ✿ Massage your legs every day for five minutes to get the blood flowing.
- ✿ Elevate your legs.
- ✿ Rest. And reduce the amount of time spent standing.
- ✿ Walking is good – contracting your calf muscles helps to pump the blood uphill through your veins and into your pelvis.
- ✿ Breathing from your diaphragm optimizes your venous system for many reasons, including pushing blood up to your brain/ pulling blood up from your legs.
- ✿ And some recipe ideas: tabbouleh (see p. 169); parsley tea (made with 1 teaspoon dried parsley per cup, steeped for a few minutes) – parsley helps the veins; nettle tea (see p. 138); leafy green vegetables and beetroot.

Other old-fashioned remedies I have heard of that I will share with you, but which may not appeal, are using raw grated potato peel directly on to the piles or a garlic clove wrapped in gauze and inserted into the rectum overnight.

Tips by type

Spleen type

Tiredness and a feeling of heaviness and lethargy in the body, as if things are dragging down and falling out of you. You have no enthusiasm for anything and no appetite for life or food. Your stool is loose and you look really pale.

Tongue: Pale and swollen.

Tips: Diet to nourish your Spleen (see p. 178). Moxa on St 36 (see p. 112).

Damp and/or Heat type

Lots of itching and swelling around the anus. Heavy protruding with bleeding of the stools. The stool may be very smelly and stick to the side of the toilet when you flush.

Tongue: Coated – normally with a white coating indicating Damp and Cold, or a yellow coating, indicating Heat.

Tips: Include lots of Damp-resolving foods in your diet (see p. 58). Avoid spicy foods, cayenne and black pepper.

CASE STUDY

THAT SINKING FEELING

Emily had come to me in her first pregnancy with very bad haemorrhoids. She was twenty weeks pregnant, and although I was able to ease her suffering a little with acupuncture and some lifestyle advice, it was really a case of 'damage limitation', the problem being quite set in and hard to reverse by the time I saw her. We did, however, stop them from getting worse, and I said that in her next pregnancy she should try to see me before this became a problem again.

Next time round, Emily dutifully came to see me at twelve weeks. The piles had started earlier this pregnancy, and she was keen that they should not develop into the problem she'd had first time around. I gave her one acupuncture treatment and Emily followed all my advice and took adequate rest. We then did acupuncture once a month throughout the rest of her pregnancy. Not only did the haemorrhoids not progress, but they disappeared altogether, never to return.

TABBOULEH

This recipe can be made with the traditional bulgur wheat or with quinoa. Parsley is an excellent Blood tonic and also drains excess fluid from the body. This is also the perfect recipe for those who are feeling a bit 'stuck' or Stagnant.

Serves 6–8

480ml (2 pints) chicken stock (see p. 254) or chicken or vegetable bouillon

170g (6oz) bulgur wheat or quinoa

1/3 cucumber, peeled, deseeded and roughly chopped

3 ripe, but firm tomatoes, peeled, deseeded and chopped

large bunch of flat-leaf parsley, finely chopped

large bunch of curly parsley, finely chopped

large bunch of mint, finely chopped

6 spring onions, or 3 small shallots, finely sliced

freshly ground black pepper, to taste

For the dressing:

juice of 2 juicy large lemons

120ml (4fl oz) olive oil

1 teaspoon sea salt

1 teaspoon ground cumin

1. Bring the stock to the boil, add the bulgur wheat or quinoa. Stir, cover and reduce to a low heat. Cook for about 15–20 minutes, stirring occasionally until plumped up (check packet instructions). Drain any excess liquid, fluff with a fork, then set aside to cool.
2. Place the cucumber and tomato in a bowl, along with the parsley, mint and onions.
3. In a jar with a lid, combine the dressing ingredients and shake vigorously until emulsified.
4. Add the bulgur wheat or quinoa to the bowl (it's fine if it's still a bit warm), add all the dressing and stir well. Season with black pepper and more

salt if needed. Let the tabbouleh sit for a couple of hours before serving, or refrigerate overnight and bring up to room temperature to serve – the flavours meld together well as it sits.

Headaches and migraine

It is not uncommon for women to experience headaches and migraine during pregnancy.

Why does it happen?

Headaches and migraines during pregnancy are often caused by muscle tension in the neck or by eyestrain. Hormonal changes can also increase the tension and sinusitis can also cause headache symptoms – that head-cold feeling (see p. 216).

Note: Severe headaches that don't go away and headaches experienced in your forehead area, intolerance to bright lights and swelling in the hands and feet may indicate pregnancy-induced hypertension or pre-eclampsia and must be reported to your midwife.

In Chinese medicine terms, headaches usually involve excessive energy rising to the head, often involving the Liver energy. In particular, headaches involving the temples are considered Liver and Gallbladder headaches and are common during pregnancy due to the general Stagnation of energy that normally affects these two organs' systems. Headaches affecting the forehead are considered digestive and those affecting the occiput (back of neck) are to do with muscular tension. Blood-Deficient headaches are often accompanied by dizziness or dots (floaters) in front of the eyes.

What can you do?

- ❀ Drink room-temperature water and herbal teas throughout the day. But don't flood your system, especially at mealtimes – drink little and often to keep well hydrated.
- ❀ If the pain is mild and you feel a little 'fuzzy', try going for a gentle walk.

❀ If you work at a computer screen, take regular breaks away from your desk and look away from the screen for a couple of minutes every quarter of an hour or so.

❀ Certain foods can be a trigger for headaches – try to avoid cheese, chocolate and too much wheat.

❀ For Liver-type headaches (temples), reduce foods that disturb the Liver energy. These are generally sour foods, such as vinegar, pickles, yogurt, grapefruit juice.

❀ Blood-Deficient headaches require rest and Blood-nourishing foods (see p. 57). These types are especially sensitive to stimulation.

❀ Dampen a cloth with cold water and wring it out. Place it over the eyes and the forehead and lie quietly breathing and imagining the cool moisture of the cloth absorbing all the excess heat and energy from your head.

❀ Acupuncture has been shown to help with headaches and migraines.[18]

EYE TREATMENTS

Sometimes, itchy or dry eyes can trigger headaches. For itchy eyes, try either nettle tea or 'palming' – rub your palms together vigorously until they generate heat, then cup your hands over your eyes for a minute. You can do this as often as you like.

For dry, red eyes, try an eye mask that you can make at home: slice a cold cucumber very thinly and put into a damp muslin cloth. Store in the fridge for a while, then lie down and place over your eyes. Or try chrysanthemum tea – drink some of the tea and then leave the rest to cool. Dampen a flat cotton pad in the cool, strained tea and use to bathe your eyes.

A good eye exercise for tired eyes is to imagine the eye as the face of a clock; start by directing your gaze at twelve on your imaginary clock, then move your eyes – using just the eye muscles – to one, then two and so on, until you have gone full circle.

Gestational diabetes

If you already have diabetes, you will have discussed this with your doctor before and during your pregnancy. It isn't common, but a small percentage of women develop diabetes in pregnancy. When it does occur, gestational diabetes usually develops in the latter half of pregnancy and goes away afterwards.

Why does it happen?

During pregnancy, your body needs to produce extra insulin and usually your hormones will trigger this. When your body doesn't produce enough insulin you can't regulate your own blood-sugar levels and diabetes develops. Factors that increase your risk of developing gestational diabetes include:

❀ a family history of the condition
❀ having had a previous baby with a birthweight of over 5.8kg
❀ being overweight or obese
❀ polycystic ovary syndrome (PCOS)
❀ being Asian, black Caribbean or Middle Eastern.

Gestational diabetes may be associated with pre-eclampsia (see p. 221), premature labour and excess amniotic fluid. You'll also be at a higher risk of developing type 2 diabetes later in life, as will your child. Your baby may be large for dates, due to the extra glucose.

Symptoms may include feeling tired, needing to go to the loo more often and increased thirst. However these may be difficult to spot as many pregnant women experience them whether they have gestational diabetes or not. If your doctor suspects you may be developing this condition, your blood sugar will be measured or a glucose-tolerance test may be performed (where you will be given a sugary drink and the blood sugar measured after one and two hours).

What can you do?

If you are diagnosed with gestational diabetes, you will be monitored carefully and given advice on diet and exercise, which matches the general advice I give all my patients:

- ❀ Eat plenty of complex carbohydrates to give a steady release of energy, including whole grains, oats, potatoes, lentils and beans.
- ❀ Eat small amounts of lean proteins.
- ❀ Eat plenty of fruit and vegetables.
- ❀ Do moderate exercise like walking for around half an hour a day.

A small number of women need insulin tablets or injections. You'll be taught to recognize the early signs of hypoglycaemia (which is when you have too much insulin), and told to keep something like a sugary drink to hand. The signs include:

- ❀ looking pale
- ❀ feeling shaky
- ❀ sweating
- ❀ feeling very hungry.

Qigong – Eight Strands of the Brocade

This is a dynamic set of exercises, often said to benefit the Lungs, Spleen and Stomach, Energy and Strength, Kidneys, Heart, Muscles, Joints and Liver, and, therefore, a wonderful overall exercise. Qigong is particularly good for the second trimester as this is a time when you can begin to get your Qi moving again and prevent Stagnation. It is balancing and gently energizing.

There are eight stances and each is repeated eight times. As you do the exercises, always try to feel centred. As you explore upwards, don't lose a sense of down, for example. Stand with feet about shoulder-width apart and parallel. Allow your body to be comfortable and don't lose balance.

1. Pressing palms to heaven
Start with the hands in front at mid-chest height, palms facing the chest and fingertips almost touching.

As you breathe in, let the hands rise in front of and past the face and twist the palms until your hands are above your head and palms face the ceiling.

As you breathe out, press the hands upwards and rise up on to your toes. Continue the movement, so that the hands (with straight arms) descend past the face (palms facing away) continuing down until they turn naturally at the bottom and rise to the start point. At the same time come back from tiptoes.

Repeat eight times.

2. Drawing the bow
In this stance, the feet are about two shoulder-widths apart, but feet are still parallel and the hips always face the front – try not to twist them. Cross your arms at the wrists, in front of the face with loose fists, palms towards you.

As you breathe in, look to the left side. The left hand straightens to the left and the right arm draws back the imaginary string of a bow. Try to keep the right hand forward of face level (don't over open the chest). Move your weight on to the right leg.

As you breathe out, gently return to the start position.

Repeat to the right and then alternate for six more.

3. Separating earth and heaven
Return to natural (feet shoulder-width apart) stance. Start with the hands in the same position as stance 1.

As you breathe in, raise one hand to the ceiling (palm to ceiling) and press the other to the ground (palm to floor).

As you breathe out return to the start position.

4. Yielding and opening to the side
Start with the arms resting by your sides. As you breathe in, raise the left arm to vertical. As you breathe out the arm continues its journey over the head and the right side of the waist yields, allowing the left to open and the body to bend.

On the next in-breath, the arm moves back to the vertical, but the body remains bent. As you breathe out, the body returns to upright as the arm comes down to the side.

Alternate on each side four times and try to sense when the body is ready to bend and return to upright.

5. Turning to gaze at the moon
The main focus of this exercise is to turn the spine. The hips stay facing forward and the knees do not really move at all.

Start in the same position as stance 1. On the in-breath, begin to turn the spine from the base, gently moving your focus up the spine as the limit of turn is reached in each stage. This is a smooth movement, and as the neck is part of the spine, your head turns too at the end of the in-breath.

On the out-breath gently unwind the spine back to the starting position. Repeat four times on each side.

6. Bending knees

Start with legs hip-width apart and arms by your side. As you breathe in, gently lift the hands (bending at the elbow) palms facing up, then turning over to face down.

As you breathe out, press your palms towards the ground and bend the knees, keeping the back straight – don't bend too far.

On the next breath, push through the soles of your feet and feel the energy lifting you, knees straightening and lower arms repeating their cycle, palms up and then turning over ready for the next out-breath.

Repeat eight times.

7. Punching

Stand with feet hip-width apart with loose fists at your waist, palms up.

On the in-breath, punch straight out with your left fist and, as you do so, tighten your muscles, starting from the feet, up the legs and buttocks, into the back and shoulders (shoulders tensing downwards not up). The fist turns over as you punch.

As you breathe out and the fist returns to the waist, let all the tension go and feel completely relaxed.

Repeat four times on alternate sides.

8. Warming the kidneys

Stand in normal stance. Place your hands on your lower-back (kidney) area and gently massage. Relaxing the shoulders completely, begin to bounce on the balls of your feet, so that the hands on your lower back move up and down, giving the kidneys a gentle massage.

As you bounce, try and be aware of breathing in and out, and let the breath be a bit broken from the bouncing.

These exercises have been kindly contributed by Simon and Sally Givertz (see Resources, p. 343, for more information).

Second-trimester Yoga

Learning to move with ease is a priority during this time, because it will stand you in good stead as your body grows larger and heavier in the later months. Yoga offers some beautiful sequences to enable you to move gracefully and fluidly through your pregnancy, allowing you to adapt your posture and ways of moving in response to the changes your body is experiencing. Always be sure to breathe easily and freely with a full yogic breath (see p. 196) as you move, synchronizing your body, breath and mind. The rhythmic flowing movements create a soothing, rocking environment for your baby to enjoy as much as you. **Note:** If you have pain in the pelvic joints, then skip step 5 completely. Simply keep both knees on the mat and raise the hips directly above them, so that you can follow the instructions for the arms from 'high kneeling'.

Sun and earth salutation for pregnancy

1. Stand in the middle of your mat, knees bent, feet at least hip-width apart or wider, if that feels more comfortable.
2. Do three or more pelvic scoops (for full instructions, see p. 164).
3. Reach your hands up above your head as you inhale.
4. Bend your knees as you fold forwards, and slowly bring your hands down to the mat, keeping the knees bent, and bringing them both down to the floor at the same time, coming on to all fours.
5. Step the right foot off the mat to the side, and rest the right elbow on the right knee. Circle the left hand, keeping the elbow bent and watching the hand moving through the air. Breathe in as the hand lifts, and out as it descends. Repeat at least three times, continuing as long as you like.
6. Keep the right foot in the same position and bring both hands to the mat in front of you, circling the hips at least three times in each direction. Inhale as you move forward and exhale as you drop back.
7. Bring the right knee back on to the mat under the hips, returning to all fours and moving the whole body in a circling action, inhaling for one half of the circle and exhaling for the other half of the circle.

8. Cat pose: inhale as the chest and head lift, keeping the lower back flat. Exhale as the back rounds, tucking the tailbone under and lengthening the curve in the lower back. Repeat at least three times.
9. Cat swoops: take the knees a little wider, and as you exhale, tuck the tailbone under, round the lower back and sink your buttocks back towards your heels. Keep your hands firmly on the mat, perhaps a little wider than before, and inhale as you bend your elbows out to the side and swoop forwards to the level of your thumbs. Straighten the arms, and then sink the buttocks back to the heels, rounding the back. Repeat at least three times.
10. Child's pose (rest for as long as you need): buttocks on to the heels (or on to a bolster, if that is more comfortable), head on the floor or on a cushion, arms resting in front of you.
11. Return to all fours and then back up to standing by pressing the palms of the hands on to the floor, lifting both the knees up as the hands pad back towards the knees, shift the weight back into the heels as you straighten up.
12. Repeat the sequence with the left foot out to the side of the mat.

This energizing and revitalizing sequence can be used throughout your pregnancy. Many of the floor-based poses are very useful during labour, so it's nice to be familiar with them. Add a bolster pillow between your heels to make these easier to do as your bump grows larger. Breathe freely with *ujayii* breath (see p. 196) as you move. Enjoy!

For more information on Uma Dinsmore-Tuli's books and website, and yoga in pregnancy, please see Resources, p. 339, and Further Reading, p. 347.

Is the Fuel Good?

If you have been feeling rotten up to this point with nausea and sickness, your appetite will probably return in the second trimester. It's the perfect time to focus on nourishing the Spleen, so that your digestion can absorb as many nutrients as possible from the food you eat. Simply eating a healthy, balanced diet will go a long way towards giving your digestion a helping hand. In addition, I have included some advice and foods below specific to building Spleen and Stomach Qi.

As well as the physical role of the Spleen in relation to digestion, in Chinese medicine we also attribute to it emotional and psychological roles. A strong Spleen lays the foundations for emotional health and the Spleen is the organ that is archetypically related to the mother, and so is responsible for our inner nurturing. Good Spleen energy creates a sense of well-being and contentment. We feel balanced, grounded and at ease with ourselves and others.

When Spleen energy is reduced there is a tendency to feel out of balance; perhaps there is too much introspection or projecting on to others. There might be little appetite for breakfast and digestion is affected. This can lead to Stagnation, so use your renewed sense of energy to keep the Spleen Qi strong.

Being good to your Spleen

- ❀ Eat a good breakfast – in Chinese medicine, Stomach energy is at its peak between 7 and 9 a.m. If you don't fancy breakfast, it is a sign of weakened Spleen energy, so it's a good idea to eat something that's easy to digest, like porridge. Other good breakfast foods include boiled, poached or scrambled eggs, fruit salad with a sprinkling of nuts or a smoothie made with yogurt, fruit and milk (for Yin deficient types).
- ❀ Grains are sweet and nourishing for the Spleen, as are root vegetables and, in particular, yellow/orange foods.
- ❀ Gentle and aromatic spices are beneficial for stimulating digestion.
- ❀ Well-cooked food is preferred to raw when it comes to building good Spleen energy.
- ❀ Try not to eat meals late at night, as this is the time when your Stomach energy is at its low point.
- ❀ Eating small meals regularly keeps the Stomach and Spleen energy balanced. Don't skip meals.
- ❀ Don't flood your digestion by drinking lots of water with your meals. Drink water and herbal teas in between meals as much as possible.
- ❀ Enjoying your food and eating when relaxed, as well as chewing slowly and savouring each mouthful all contribute to Spleen Qi, as your body is focused on the food and digestion, rather than, say, working or reading at the same time.

❀ Try not to be overly concerned about your diet or indeed anything
  – stay balanced and relaxed, and ask for any support if you need it.

Store cupboard for the second trimester
Foods to nourish the Spleen:

❀ Grains – barley, oats, rice, rye, spelt
❀ Root vegetables – carrots, parsnips, pumpkin, squash, sweet
  potatoes
❀ Orange/yellow foods – carrots, pepper, pumpkin, red lentils,
  squash, sweet potatoes
❀ Aromatic herbs and spices – cardamom, cinnamon, fennel seeds,
  garlic, ginger, marjoram, sage, thyme, turmeric

Sweet Potato and Lentil Soup
This is a wonderfully warming and nourishing soup. The Stomach likes the
moistness and natural sweetness. Ginger and cinnamon warm and open
the channels, while lentils boost the Qi and coconut milk is good for the
Heart. (**Note:** not good for Heat.)

Serves 6–8
2 tablespoons olive oil
1 large onion, chopped
1kg (2lb 2oz) sweet potatoes, peeled and chopped into chunks
2 teaspoons ground cinnamon
½ teaspoon paprika
1 tablespoon fresh root ginger, peeled and chopped
125g (4½oz) organic split red lentils, rinsed and drained
1 litre (1¾ pints) boiling water, mixed with 4 teaspoons vegetarian
  bouillon stock
200ml (7fl oz) organic coconut milk
salt and pepper

1. Heat the oil in a large saucepan over medium heat. Add the onion and fry for 5–10 minutes or until translucent and soft without browning.
2. Add the sweet potato pieces, then the cinnamon, paprika and ginger. Stir to coat the sweet potato with the spices and onion. Cover with a lid and leave for 5 minutes.
3. Add the lentils and stock to the saucepan. Bring to the boil, then reduce the heat and simmer for 30 minutes.
4. Remove soup from the heat, transfer to a blender and whizz until smooth.
5. Leave to cool for 5 minutes, then add the coconut milk before giving it one last quick whizz to blend.
6. Add salt and pepper to taste before serving.

Lamb Hotpot

This is not called a hotpot for nothing! This recipe is warming in every way – call it central heating for the body. Lamb is the most heating of all the meats, and thyme and rosemary the most heating of herbs, making this a wonderful recipe to raise the Yang of the body. Red wine too is warm and robust in nature, bringing a deep, satisfying warmth to this recipe to heat up even the chilliest evening.

Serves 4
450g (1lb) lamb, diced into 2.5cm (1in) cubes
salt and freshly ground pepper, to taste
20g (¾oz) flour
120ml (4fl oz) oil
30g (1oz) butter
150g (5½oz) chestnut mushrooms, sliced
2 medium onions, diced
3 garlic cloves, peeled and sliced
2 tablespoons fresh thyme leaves
½ teaspoon sugar

2 sprigs fresh rosemary
240ml (8fl oz) beef or chicken stock
240ml (8fl oz) red wine
5 large potatoes

1. Preheat the oven to 180°C/350°F/gas mark 4.
2. Place the lamb pieces in a mixing bowl, adding salt and pepper and the flour. Make sure each piece is coated in flour.
3. Put the oil in a large saucepan, over medium heat. When hot, add the lamb pieces for browning – turn with tongs to brown on all sides; this should take about 5 minutes. Take off the heat, remove the lamb from the saucepan and set aside.
4. Return the pan to the heat (medium–high) and add half the butter and the mushrooms. Season, then let them brown, for about 5 minutes. Add the diced onions, garlic, thyme and sugar and the leaves from one of the sprigs of rosemary. Reduce the heat and let the onions caramelize for about 5–7 minutes, stirring occasionally.
5. Return the lamb to the saucepan, turn the heat up again and add the stock and wine, bringing everything to a simmer for 10 minutes or so, before turning off the heat.
6. While the lamb is simmering, peel and thinly slice the potatoes.
7. Using a casserole or oven dish (greased with oil or butter) add a layer of potatoes and season. Spoon a layer of the lamb mixture on top, followed by another layer of potatoes, season again. Add the rest of the lamb and sauce followed by the last layer of potatoes. Season again, and dot little pieces of the remaining butter generously over the potatoes. Add the second sprig of rosemary in the middle for decoration and place in the preheated oven for 2 hours.

Warm and Spicy Rice Pudding

A warming and Yin-nourishing dish, perfect for Yin/Yang balance. This is also delicious in hot weather after being chilled in the fridge for a couple of hours. (**Note:** not good for Damp.)

Serves 2

600ml (20fl oz) milk
3 cloves
1 teaspoon ground ginger
½ teaspoon ground cardamom
¼ teaspoon ground cinnamon
4 level tablespoons maple or agave syrup
8 heaped tablespoons Arborio risotto rice

1. Heat the milk over a high heat, then stir in all the other ingredients.
2. When the mixture begins to boil, reduce to a very low simmer, give it a stir and cover the saucepan with a lid.
3. Keep an eye on the mixture for about 20 minutes or until the rice is cooked and it looks like rice pudding, stirring every now and then.
4. Turn off the heat and let it sit for another 20 minutes, before removing the cloves and serving.

Foods to nourish Yin

Women in pregnancy often tend to be a little out of balance in terms of Yin or Yang. As discussed earlier, in the 360-degree health check, signs of Yin Deficiency include Five Palm Heat, where you have heat or mild sweating in the palms of your hands or soles of your feet, a feeling of heat in the centre of the chest, night sweats, feeling hot in the afternoon, dry skin and feelings of anxiety. In these cases, foods to include are:

❀ Grains: barley, millet, spelt, wheat
❀ Vegetables: artichokes, potatoes, string beans, sweet potatoes, yams

- ❀ Fruit: apricots, avocados, bananas, mangoes, pears, pineapple, plums, pomegranate, strawberries
- ❀ Pulses: black beans, kidney beans, black soybeans, tofu
- ❀ Nuts and seeds: coconut milk, flaxseeds (linseeds), pine kernels, black and white sesame seeds
- ❀ Fish: mullet, sardines (limit to 2 portions a week)
- ❀ Meat/dairy: beef, duck, goose, pork, rabbit, butter, cheese, eggs, milk (cow or goat), yogurt
- ❀ Herbs and spices: nettle
- ❀ Condiments: sesame oil, honey

Sesame Seed Banana Bread

The moistening action of the bananas, sesame seeds and agave syrup make this a wonderful Yin-nourishing recipe. The allspice and cinnamon have a gentle warming function, bringing some balance to the recipe and they offset some of its dampening qualities. Sadly, not enough to make this suitable for truly Damp conditions who should avoid it.

Dry ingredients:
115g (4oz) organic white rice flour
170g (6oz) chickpea (garbanzo bean) flour
2 level teaspoons baking powder
1 level teaspoon bicarbonate of soda
1 teaspoon allspice
½ teaspoon cinnamon
½ teaspoon sea salt

Wet ingredients:
115g (4oz) butter (room temperature), plus a little extra for greasing
180ml (6fl oz) agave syrup or 200g (7oz) sugar
2 extra-large eggs
2 tablespoons milk (organic goat's milk works well)

Other ingredients:
3 very ripe bananas
40g (1¼oz) sesame seeds
2 tablespoons lemon juice
2 tablespoons agave syrup (or 3 tablespoons sugar)
1 or 2 tablespoons boiling water (1 if using agave; 2 if using sugar)

1. Preheat the oven to 180°C/350°F/gas mark 4 and grease and line a 25 x 13cm (10 x 5in) loaf tin with parchment paper.
2. Sift all the dry ingredients into a large mixing bowl and set aside.
3. In another large mixing bowl, cut the butter into small cubes and set it aside for a few minutes while you prepare the bananas. Peel the bananas and slice them on to a large plate. Using a fork, lightly mash each slice – leaving some bigger pieces; this will result in nice chunky pieces of banana throughout the bread.
4. Using a wooden spoon, cream the butter and add the agave syrup, until the butter pales in colour and the consistency is light and smooth and creamy. Gradually add in each egg, followed by the milk. Add the bananas to the wet ingredients, stirring lightly.
5. Fold in the dry ingredients, adding a little at a time until it is all combined. No need to overwork the batter – a light touch here will keep more air in the batter, giving a fluffier texture to the finished bread. Add the sesame seeds to the mixture, reserving some to sprinkle on top of the batter before baking.
6. Pour the mixture into the prepared tin, sprinkle with the reserved seeds and bake in the preheated oven for 50 minutes. Reduce the temperature to 160°C/325°F/gas mark 3 and bake for a further 20 minutes, keeping an eye on it. The bread is ready when a knife or skewer inserted into the middle of the loaf comes out clean. Remove from the oven, remove the parchment and let it cool on a rack for at least 20 minutes.
7. Combine the lemon juice, agave syrup and hot water in a little bowl or cup. (If you are using sugar, heat in a small saucepan on the cooker, stirring until all the sugar is dissolved.)

8. Using a cocktail stick or skewer, make tiny holes across the surface of your loaf and drizzle the lemony syrup all over it. Let it sit for another 30 minutes.
9. Serve in slices with seasonal fresh fruit for breakfast, or with ice cream, crème fraîche or whipped cream and berries for dessert.

Foods to nourish Yang

Yang is the activating force in the body, so if you are feeling as if you have no get-up-and-go at all and tend towards feeling cold and lethargic, you may feel the benefit of Yang-nourishing foods. (This applies towards the end of pregnancy especially, where the body moves from the Yin phase of pregnancy into the Yang phase of birth.) Garlic is a particularly Yang-nourishing food and others include:

- ❀ Grains: quinoa
- ❀ Nuts: chestnut, walnuts
- ❀ Fish: anchovies, trout (limit to 2 portions a week)
- ❀ Meat/dairy: beef kidney, lamb, lamb kidney, mutton, venison
- ❀ Herbs and spices: basil, rosemary, cardamom, cinnamon

Roasted Onion and Garlic Jam

This can be served warm, at room temperature or cold, with meats or vegetables, as a relish with bread and cheese or as the filling for a simple tart. It will keep in an airtight container in the fridge for up to a month.

Makes about 1 jar

60ml (2fl oz) olive oil
60ml (2fl oz) red wine
60ml (2fl oz) balsamic vinegar
1–2 teaspoons brown sugar (optional, depending on taste and sweetness of the balsamic you are using)
2 teaspoons dried rosemary, or 2 fresh sprigs, 8–10cm (3–4in) in length

1½ teaspoons Maldon salt
½ teaspoon ground cinnamon
½ teaspoon red-chilli pepper flakes (optional)
2 medium red onions, diced
1 medium yellow onion, diced
10–15 medium garlic cloves, peeled and cut in half
juice of ½ juicy lemon

1. Preheat the oven to 220°C/425°F/gas mark 7.
2. In a medium-sized casserole dish with a lid, put the olive oil, red wine, balsamic vinegar, sugar (if using), rosemary, salt, cinnamon and chilli flakes (if using). Add the onions and place in the preheated oven, *covered*, for 30 minutes.
3. Remove from the oven, add the garlic, squeeze over the lemon juice and replace in the oven, *uncovered*, for another hour.
4. Remove from the oven, give the mixture a good stir and make sure there is enough liquid – it should still be quite runny. If not add 60–120ml (2–4fl oz) water. Try to ensure that all the pieces are covered with liquid, so they don't dry out. Return to the oven, *uncovered*, for another 15 minutes.
5. Repeat the previous step, but without adding any more water – it should be reducing and getting thicker.
6. After 15 minutes repeat the process again, this time tasting for seasoning, stirring well and checking the consistency – it should be getting quite jammy now. With the back of the spoon, lightly crush the garlic pieces and stir them in, then replace the lid and return to the oven for the last 30 minutes, *covered*.
7. Remove from the oven and allow to cool. If you used fresh rosemary sprigs, remove them now.

Ideas for meals

Where I have suggested a salad, eat it with a soup on all but the warmest of summer days.

Yin-nourishing

- ❀ Salad of alfalfa sprouts, avocado, string beans, asparagus
- ❀ Three-bean salad – choose your favourite three beans and add olive oil, lime juice and black sesame seeds
- ❀ Poached egg and asparagus
- ❀ Baked potato with grated cheese
- ❀ Sardines on toast
- ❀ Crab and avocado (crab must be cooked and cooled properly; to be on the safe side, best to eat it only if you've cooked it yourself)
- ❀ Snacks: apricots, pineapple, watermelon, bananas and mango; bars made from black and white sesame seeds, honey and walnuts
- ❀ Nettle tea
- ❀ Coconut milk or water

Yang-nourishing

- ❀ Stir-fried chicken and ginger
- ❀ Quinoa and thyme salad
- ❀ Oven-roasted vegetables with garlic and rosemary
- ❀ Risotto of chestnuts and butternut squash
- ❀ Leek and potato soup
- ❀ Snacks: pine nuts, pistachio nuts, cherries, raspberries, peaches
- ❀ Tea: thyme, jasmine, ginger, cinnamon

Is the Mind on Board?

In the second trimester, the emphasis is on keeping a healthy balance. Go out and enjoy yourself, but still take care and time to relax and rest as well. If you are stressed out and working all hours, it will affect your unborn baby, and long-term stress can also cause tiredness, depression and make you more vulnerable to illness. So look after your Heart, the home of your emotions.

Rituals and the Heart

I think we have forgotten the power of rituals and see them in a rather negative light, perhaps as slightly weird or religious. But rituals have always been a part of human life and in societies where people still live more traditionally, they play an important role. In Chinese medicine, rituals are very good for the Heart and give us a sense of being part of a greater order.

I have some rituals at work that I use to prepare myself for the challenges of a full day of practice, when there is no knowing what might come my way. I have some items that are precious to me and remind me of people and some items that I feel offer me protection. I fill a beautiful jug with fresh water and think about the many women who have to walk miles every day to collect clean water for themselves and their family. I think that water is a wonderful female symbol and without water there is no life. In Chinese medicine, it also represents the Kidney energy, which is an important part of our work with fertility and pregnancy. I silently thank every patient for entrusting me with their health. These are simple things, but they remind me of how blessed we are and it helps me tune into my patients' needs. It also highlights that we are not alone in the world and that we are part of a bigger picture.

CASE STUDY

PATCHWORK QUEEN

A patient of mine who was normally more comfortable holding court in the boardroom discovered a hidden skill during her pregnancy.

Restless and agitated in the evenings, and not wanting to watch television, think about work or use the computer, she decided to make a patchwork quilt for her baby. She asked her mum and her sisters to send her scraps of material from old dresses and other items from her childhood. Having grown up in the 1970s, she amassed quite a collection, and soon became inspired by the snippets of her past: her first party dress, the favourite old Liberty-print dress, those purple pincord trousers she had worn to death, her mother's highly patterned party dress (she remembered her looking like a princess in it) and even the softest piece of fabric from a once-loved nightdress.

Night after night, she stitched these precious bits of memory on to squares of cardboard, then patiently stitched these together in long lines of random colours and patterns. It became a labour of love, and just a week before she gave birth the masterpiece was completed.

She said it was one of the things she had achieved in her life that she was most proud of (this woman was CEO of a successful company). Not only had it reminded her of where she came from and the importance of her own family, but it had helped her to relax and switch off in the evenings. The repetitive action of the sewing was exactly the right activity to oppose the very cerebral job she had in the day. The reward was a stunning quilt for her new baby, full of family memories.

Dreams during pregnancy

If your dreams do not disturb the sleep, are not frightening and do not stay with you the next day, making you feel unsettled, then they are considered normal. However, if they are excessive, in that they cause your sleep to be disturbed, or they are nightmares, then this is seen as an imbalance in Chinese medicine.

Yin and Blood Deficiency

Excessive dreaming often with night sweating. Don't get over-stimulated before bedtime or watch too much TV or use the computer. Make sure your food contains lots of Blood-nourishing foods (see p. 57) and don't eat late at night.

Phlegm and Heat

Restless dreams and feeling hot and congested. Make sure you don't eat cheese before bedtime. This is an old-fashioned piece of advice, but it makes sense in Chinese medicine. If the digestion is churning away at night, trying to digest that lump of cheese, it stands to reason that the mind will be disturbed and keep thoughts churning around in your head.

Heart/mind

Dreams which wake you up. Practise night-time rituals and relax in a bath with a candle burning. Meditate and find some space for calmness before bed.

SPECIAL-PLACE VISUALIZATION – TO PRACTISE THROUGHOUT PREGNANCY AND BIRTH
(from Emma Roberts)

I'd like you to create a special place in your mind – a place you can go to whenever you want to relax and enjoy a deeper level of comfort, both while you are pregnant and during the birth. Soon, you will become an expert at relaxing, and will be able to do so at any time.

Think of a place (either real or imaginary) you have been to or would like to visit. If you think of more than one place, choose one that is most appropriate for right now.

Now, while you are in this special place, I'd like you to notice everything around you. Notice the colours – how bright or pale they are – notice any sounds and any smells there might be. Notice too how your body is responding to this special place – the sensations and temperature of the air on your skin, and what feelings and thoughts are invoked by being there. Take time to just relax and enjoy the space around you. Just do what you need to do to make it completely perfect.

While you are in your special place, I'd like you to reach down into your womb and meet your growing baby. Touch and caress it, share with it the love and tenderness within you and let it know just how special it is. Reassure your baby that it is totally loved there, inside you, and that it too can relax with you and allow itself to take whatever nutrients it needs to continue growing bigger and stronger every minute.

Now take your baby by the hand and show it your special place. While you are doing this, you can talk to your baby, telling it about yourself and your life and how much you are looking forward to its birth, when the time is healthy and right for you both to meet. Enjoy this time alone with your growing baby inside you, sharing this very special place, knowing that this is somewhere you can both return to and enjoy at any time.

And now allow your baby to return to your womb, warmly and comfortably until the time is right for it to be born.

Know that this special, safe place is somewhere you can visit at any time during your pregnancy, labour and birth, and that every time you return to it, you will go into it even more quickly and deeply than the time before.

During labour, as you feel a contraction beginning and return to this special place, the contraction will be experienced only as pressure and tightening, with you knowing that each time you feel these sensations, you are nearer the moment when you will finally meet your baby. In fact, you can welcome and embrace each contraction as it comes, knowing it is positive and natural and that you have the tools to manage this birth in exactly the way you want to. You will always be aware of what is going on around you and will be able to follow instructions and answer questions, but your focus will remain with your body and your baby and what you are in the process of achieving, as you give birth easily and calmly and naturally.

Thank your unconscious mind for helping you to create this special place and for allowing you to take whatever it is you needed to learn from this experience.

Common Conditions

Snoring
Many pregnant women complain about snoring during pregnancy.

Why does it happen?
It is due to the excess Phlegm in the system, and usually comes from a faulty digestive system or one that is under strain.

What can you do?
Follow the principles of keeping your digestive system healthy and avoid foods that overburden it. If the snoring is becoming a problem, try to eliminate Phlegm-forming foods (see p. 217) and don't eat late at night. If the body is still struggling to digest dinner when you are meant to be sleeping, it will have a difficult job and this may well cause your sleep and breathing to become laboured.

Restless legs and cramps
Cramps most often occur deep in the calf muscles and can be really painful. Restless legs can become very jumpy late in the evening and can keep you awake at night, making this a particularly frustrating pregnancy ailment.

Why does it happen?

It is not known why this happens, although dehydration is thought to be a possible cause. In Chinese medicine, they are generally considered to be the result of Stagnation of energy.

What can you do?

- ❀ Stretch out the calf muscle by straightening the leg and flexing the toes to stretch out the channel running down the back of the leg.
- ❀ Take Epsom-salt baths (see p. 70).
- ❀ Ask your GP to check your vitamin B12 levels.
- ❀ Drink plenty of fluids.

Yoga for restless legs and cramps

Yoga tip: breathe into the cramp, keep open and free.

Practice: warrior against the wall

Yoga offers some helpful preventive practices that you can also use to relieve both cramps and restless legs.

A really full yoga breath is the key to effective use of these remedies, so be sure you are breathing easily and fully, preferably allowing the breath to exit through the mouth.

Stand facing a clear space of wall, with your feet hip-width apart and toes about a metre away from the wall. Place the palms of both hands on to the wall in front of you at shoulder height and width, spreading the fingers well. Step back with your right foot, taking an easy stride and bending your left knee. Keep the right leg straight, and press the outside edge of your right heel down into the floor as you push the heels of your hands into the wall and breathe out. Breathe in softly, and each time you exhale, press the heels of the hands firmly into the wall and the heel of the right foot into the floor. Repeat for up to two minutes, consciously sending your breath down the straight leg to free the flow of energy through the site of the cramping. Pause, then, keeping your feet in the same positions, simply swap the bend in the knees, so that the right knee bends and the left one straightens. Repeat the breathing and pressing of the hands and feet in this position for up to two minutes. Then swap the feet positions, bringing the left foot back and the right foot forward and repeat the whole sequence on that side, breathing fully and freely for up to two minutes in each position.

This remedy works best if you carry the mind along with the breath, to clear the tightness and cramping along the length of the legs with each exhalation.

For more information on Uma Dinsmore-Tuli's books and website, and yoga in pregnancy, please see Resources, p. 339, and Further Reading, p. 347.

Insomnia

You may well have never had problems sleeping before but suddenly now, just when you feel you need even more sleep, you are struggling.

Why does it happen?

Insomnia in pregnancy could be due to sickness and nausea or to being uncomfortable. Sometimes, it's simply all the getting up to go to the loo in the middle of the night. Towards the end of pregnancy, the most common reasons are discomfort or heartburn.

I also think that your body is cleverly preparing you for the job in hand; when your baby arrives there will be lots of waking in the middle of the night. Your growing baby inside you probably already has its own sleep pattern which may indicate how it will be on arrival. I personally believe that it is normal for your own sleep patterns to become lighter in preparation and as a protection instinct to care and look after your new baby.

What can you do?

My advice is to try not to fight it. If you find you are sleeping less at night, try and nap in the day. I know it's hard to fit this in at work, but I also believe that employers (and I am one) need to be flexible and understanding, and half an hour with your head down on the desk is going to pay dividends to everyone in the long run. This is not a competition to see who can carry on as normal for the longest.

Tips for all

- ✿ Try a few drops of lavender oil in the bath and a five-minute massage before bed concentrating on Kid 1 (see p. 271).
- ✿ If you spend all day in front of a computer and do lots of thinking work, your brain is going to be pretty active and stimulated. If you can, offset this by walking home from work or doing something very physically relaxing that allows you to switch off.
- ✿ The mind, the Heart and the Womb are all linked in Chinese medicine, and so a calm and centred mind and a Heart that is grounded and settled will transfer calmness and peace to the Womb, and hence your baby. Address emotional issues that may have bothered you for years. I don't mean you should have a big family showdown, but I believe it is a time of peace and forgiveness and a time to let go of issues that may have held you back for years. It can be very healing, and many women are closer to their emotions now than at any other point in their lives.
- ✿ Talk to your partner and explore how you both feel about becoming parents. Share your thoughts and ideas with each other; your fears as well as your dreams. I think for many women, and for men too, it is a time of mixed emotions; on the one hand, you may feel elated about being pregnant, but on the other, afraid that you will lose something of yourself or your life with your partner. Such thoughts are normal and it is only when people become stuck on one negative thought pattern that it is a problem. (For information on help with this, see Resources, p. 339 or ask your midwife.)
- ✿ Practise calming activities like yoga, tai chi, qigong and meditation. You don't need to be able to sit for hours contemplating your navel, but it is good to be able to switch off. There are going to be times as a mother when you will need to access a deep inner calmness inside yourself when all about you is in chaos – practising now will serve you very well.
- ✿ Drink milk warmed with cardamom.

Tips by type

Let's go over some basics that might help you:

Blood Deficiency

Difficulty getting to sleep and generally feeling anxious and absent-minded. You may have palpitations. Sometimes this pattern can include digestive problems as well (but not necessarily), including poor appetite and feeling uncomfortable in the area above your navel and below your ribcage (epigastrium).

Tongue: Pale or pale and swollen.

Treatment: You need to calm down and slow down, ideally get some rest in the afternoon and, if you can't do that, when you get home from work. Put your head down on your desk or lie on your bed for thirty minutes when you get in. You don't need to sleep, but research suggests that thirty minutes' rest in the afternoon actually helps with insomnia. As my mum always said to me, 'Sleep makes sleep.' You also need to eat nourishing foods and, if you are having digestive problems, take special note of 'Being good to your Spleen' (see p. 178).

Heart Heat type

This describes a slightly more advanced sleep problem that might have started as above and has now progressed. This is why it is so important to address problems in their infancy and not let them become more entrenched.

You will be having difficulty both falling asleep and remaining asleep, and feeling very unsettled and anxious. Even when you do sleep it is fitful and full of dreams. You may also be feeling hotter than normal and may be sweating at night.

Tongue: May be red or may look as if the coating has been scraped off in an area.

Treatment: You need to switch off; you are overstimulated. Maybe you work with computers all day or in an air-conditioned office. You are always on the go and juggling a hundred different things. Cool down and find time to calm the mind. Meditation is probably the last thing you want to do, but it's what you need – or at least some time every day spent without stimulus. I have noticed that even television can be stimulating for some pregnant women if they watch it in the evening, and certainly I would ban computers after 8 p.m. and have no electrical equipment in the bedroom.

Liver Heat type

This type of insomnia will have you waking in the early hours of the morning unable to get back to sleep. Your head may be filled with thoughts and you feel irritable and agitated. For some reason, you feel unable to let go of things and you have many frustrations. You may also be sighing a great deal and have a feeling of heat in the chest. You may have headaches at the temples.

Tongue: Red, and possibly more so on the sides.

Treatment: Everything is rising to your head, which is causing the headaches and the insomnia. You might be someone who wants everything to be 'just so' and be brilliant at work, not letting anything slip. But it's time to go easy on yourself and stop trying to be in control all the time. I often ask my patients, 'What is so good about control anyway?' Ask yourself if control really is the be-all and end-all, and if it's serving you now.

Yoga for exhaustion/insomnia/breathlessness

Yoga tip: every breath makes a difference.

Practice: full yogic breath with *ujayii*

Give yourself permission to take just ten minutes to breathe well. The breath is the vehicle of *prana*, Qi, so if you pay attention to every breath, then you can bring more energy into yourself. First, get really comfortable by lying down on your mat, on your back with your knees bent and supported by a bolster. (In the later stages of pregnancy, you may be more comfortable over on your side with one knee supported by a bolster.) Dim the lights, or use a yoga eye pillow. Rest your head on a pillow, and have a blanket to cover you (especially your feet) because if you're not warm enough you won't be able to relax.

> Yawn long and loud about seven times. Release your jaw. Then settle into stillness and let your breath come and go easily through the nose. Encourage each breath out to be a total release. If it is easier for you, let the breath leave through the lips. The main thing is to feel that your whole body is breathing. When the breath comes in, feel the movements in your body to welcome the vitality which the breath brings: feel expansion sideways in the chest as the ribs move out, and movement between the shoulder blades too, enabling you to direct the breath right into your back. If there is room for your belly to

move (probably up until the twenty-eighth week this is a possibility, but after that the baby may have taken up most of the space) then allow the belly to swell and rise as you inhale, and sink down as you exhale. Don't force anything, but be fully aware of each and every breath. Let the inhalation bring vitality and energy to every cell of your body, and your baby too. Let your exhalation release you both down into a deep place of healing rest. Notice every breath. Go at whatever pace feels comfortable. When there is an easy rhythm, open your lips and let the out-breath make the sound 'Haaaaaa', so that you feel the sound in your throat like a very soft rasp. Then close your lips and make that same sound again, this time feeling how the sound stays inside the throat, like the start of a very soft little snore.

Alternate the 'Haaaaa' sound with the lips open, and then with the lips closed a couple more times, until you can feel the sound, soft and even in the throat. Then keep the lips closed and continue to breathe with this sound in the throat, both on the breath in and the breath out. It feels as if you are breathing straight through the throat. The pace of breath will probably slow.

Notice the difference after ten minutes, and use this mindful breathing whenever you are feeling tired. If you use it at night, it can help you to settle into sleep; if you use it during the day, it will calm and energize you. Every breath makes a difference.

For more information on Uma Dinsmore-Tuli's books and website, and yoga in pregnancy, please see Resources, p. 339, and Further Reading, p. 347.

CASE STUDY

PHYSICIAN HEAL THYSELF

Claire worked long hours as a doctor. She was newly qualified and had just completed a long stint on a busy accident-and-emergency ward.

She came to me in the second trimester, wanting to learn how to unwind and switch off. Working in A and E during her early pregnancy she saw many people, some of whom were in life-threatening situations, and the images often stayed with her. She felt haunted by some of what she had seen and would ruminate over people she felt she could have helped more. It was really bringing her down.

Working shifts is hard on the system and, over the years, I have seen many patients whose health has suffered due to their working life. It is important for these people to try and find ways to build in some regularity into their lives. The Spleen, in particular, likes regularity, and anything that damages the Spleen damages the digestion. On an emotional level, this can lead to rumination and an inability to absorb ideas and images. I felt this was central to Claire's problem – at a time when her body was adjusting to the huge, new challenge of her pregnancy, it (and her mind) was also having to deal with the challenge of shift work in a busy A and E ward.

We decided that she would benefit from some regular acupuncture for a few weeks, and that meditation was a good tool for her to learn herself, so she could find her own way to switch off. The idea of meditating was quite difficult for Claire, who had learnt her whole life that she could achieve things through 'doing'. The idea that *not doing* could be of benefit was a hard concept for her to grasp, but she knew she needed to find a new way to calm her system down and she was very open to trying it.

Claire taught herself to meditate. Each evening and each morning she sat in a chair and spent time following a simple meditation I had shown her; closing her eyes, taking some deep breaths and repeating 'Om' several times. Then, focusing her inner gaze to her third eye (between her two actual eyes), she would sit breathing like this for some moments, letting any thoughts leave her mind as quickly as they entered, and not dwelling on any one thought. She was very quickly able to do this for twenty minutes.

This simple meditation and Claire's will to find a way to help herself changed her life. She said that many people commented on the change in her and her inner calm and serenity. They put it down to the glow of pregnancy, and although this was the catalyst, she felt that learning to meditate was one of the most valuable things she had ever done. 'I have spent my whole life busying myself doing and achieving,' she said, 'and I had absolutely no idea so much could be achieved by simply *being*.'

Milk-poached Cod with Fennel and Dill

Milk is an age-old remedy to induce sleep, but I feel it needs the added ingredients of the fennel seeds to make it more digestible. This is a lovely, light recipe that will calm and soothe you to sleep (eat at least three hours before retiring).

Serves 4

olive oil
4 garlic cloves, peeled and crushed
1 medium red onion, diced
4 celery stalks, chopped
1 fennel bulb, sliced finely
¼ teaspoon dried thyme
½ teaspoon fennel seeds
freshly ground black pepper and sea salt
700ml (1¼ pints) milk
685g (1½lb) cod fillets
large handful of fresh dill

1. Pour a couple of glugs of olive oil into a large saucepan or stockpot (with a lid) and heat gently. Add the garlic and onion.
2. Add the celery and fennel, and cook until the onions are translucent and the celery is soft. Add the thyme, fennel seeds and seasoning.
3. Heat the milk in a separate saucepan without bringing it to the boil, then pour over the vegetables.
4. Cut the cod fillets into big chunks or strips and place them over the top of the mixture. Roughly chop the dill and add on top. Put the lid on and let it simmer over low heat for 10–12 minutes. Remove the lid after 10 minutes and give it a stir – test a piece of fish to see if it is opaque and cooked through.
5. Serve with buttery, minty new potatoes in the spring and summer and creamy, cheesy mashed potatoes in the autumn and winter.

chapter eleven
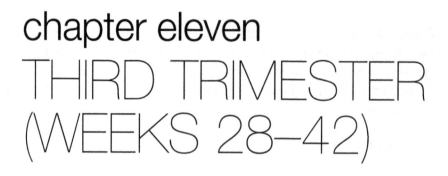
THIRD TRIMESTER (WEEKS 28–42)

The third trimester is a time of preparation and nesting; it's amazing how many couples seem to move house in the last months of pregnancy. As your bump grows, your energy and mood may swing as both your body and mind are working overtime for your developing baby. Emotional swings are normal, as most women are both excited and apprehensive about labour and also becoming a mother. Although common physical conditions like oedema and heartburn can also make life pretty uncomfortable, there is much you can do to alleviate the symptoms. This is a time to nurture and to conserve your energy as you plan for birth and beyond.

Is the Engine Working?

Throughout the third trimester, your baby grows in strength and at an amazing rate.

How your baby develops

The lungs continue to develop and mature, making breathing movements (even though they can't actually take in air until birth). The eyes will begin to open and close and distinguish between light and dark, more fine hair is growing, fingernails develop and teeth may begin to grow beneath the gums. At twenty-nine weeks, your baby is still only around one third of what the birthweight will be, around eleven weeks later.

Fat stores are laid down during the third trimester, in preparation for birth, and your baby grows at a rate of around 1cm every week. You may begin to recognize when your baby is awake or sleeping, as babies develop a pattern and yours might be moving pretty vigorously when awake. By week 36, most babies will be head down and, if this is your first pregnancy, may have descended into the pelvic girdle and become 'engaged'. Most babies will arrive in week 40, but only around 5 per cent arrive on their due date and first pregnancies often go a little overdue.

CHINESE MEDICINE AND THE THIRD TRIMESTER

In Chinese medicine, the emphasis in the third trimester is on protecting your energy, especially the Lung energy, and preparing your body and mind for labour and motherhood. You may even begin to feel very warm as your internal furnace prepares for the last few months of pregnancy and birth and increases your metabolism. It is really important to focus on the job ahead and give yourself time, so get the painters and decorators in early, as even from a practical point of view, you want to clear the house of paint fumes well before you bring your baby home. Start to think about saving your energy, take good care of yourself and act as if it is winter, keeping warm and dry and away from damp.

The Lungs are particularly susceptible to the effects of Cold towards the end of pregnancy. It might sound old-fashioned to have to dry your hair and keep warm after swimming, but I suggest this in order to protect the Lung energy for the enormous task ahead. The rhythm of the breath is going to help you through your birth and you need to protect the Lungs, so they are strong enough to do their job well. I often see women who pick up colds during the third trimester and they have real trouble shifting them for the remainder of their pregnancy. Many of the common conditions associated with the later months of pregnancy are also Damp-related, including oedema (see p. 211), sinusitis (see p. 216) and carpal-tunnel syndrome (see p. 219).

You may experience intense mood swings during the third trimester – at times, confident and elated at the prospect of becoming a mother, while at others tired, achy and apprehensive. Being fearful is human and shows how much you deeply care. But there are ways in which you can use these weeks to harmonize the Heart as you make your mental preparations. Rest, be calm as much as possible and feather the nest! Set time aside to focus on the task ahead, rather than letting yourself fall into worrying about it all day long.

A WORD FOR PARTNERS

Interestingly, in Chinese medicine the Lungs are related to the father and reflect the fact it is your role to teach your child self-value and good personal boundaries. The Lungs are also related to 'defensive' energy, and many fathers I know like to think of themselves as something of a protective shield, both for their partner and child. Yang, also masculine in nature, protects the feminine Yin, so perhaps begin to embrace this natural and possibly quite new role. Find your own strength as a parent through commitment and sustainability.

Antenatal Check-ups

From twenty-eight weeks, antenatal visits become more frequent – up to once a fortnight under thirty-six weeks, then once a week, depending on the individual circumstances of your pregnancy.

Antenatal Classes

Your local hospital or GP surgery is likely to offer free antenatal classes and women usually start attending these around week 30 of pregnancy. They are especially helpful for first-time mothers, not least because they meet other mums-to-be in their area; and often, antenatal groups continue to offer friendly postnatal support. The classes are also a useful place where you can ask any questions that you haven't been able to cover during your antenatal check-ups, which are often taken up with tests and leave little time for chatting.

The NCT (National Childbirth Trust) also offers courses all over the country, and often at times more helpful to working parents-to-be (see Resources, p. 341). You have to pay for these courses, so ask around and see what sounds right for you, as they might well differ quite a bit in terms of tone and what's included. If you are enjoying the yoga in this book you might look for a class on yoga and birth, for example.

Generally, antenatal or parentcraft courses will cover:

✿ preparation for labour, including recognizing the start of labour, relaxation techniques, breathing, when to go to hospital and forms of assisted delivery that might be needed
✿ pain relief during labour
✿ delivery of the placenta
✿ stitches
✿ care for your newborn
✿ feeding your baby
✿ postnatal recovery.

Exercise

Swimming is wonderful at this stage, giving your body much needed rest and support. Doing gentle front crawl or backstroke helps to ease the tension across your neck and shoulders, keeping your legs long, and kicking facilitates the pelvis to remain mobile and dynamic, encouraging blood supply and nurturing those tired muscles. Your baby will love this, and you will both reap the benefits.

Note: No breaststroke.

Third-trimester yoga

During the third trimester, it is delicious to be able to move freely, but more slowly, to maximize your breath and energy as you prepare for birth. Take the time to explore these movements from all fours, and set up your cushions, blankets, bolsters, chair or birthing ball for support, so that you can alternate movements with well-supported rest. These cat-pose movements with breath are all helpful ways to keep mobile, energized and comfortable in pregnancy, but have the special benefit of encouraging the baby into an optimal foetal position (head down, spine resting over to the left side of the belly), as well as being useful labour and birthing positions too.

Reconnecting with the breath

Before you start, take a moment to reconnect with the easy flow of *ujayii* breath (for full explanation, see p. 196), feeling the soft rasping feeling in your throat as the breath enters and leaves. Notice the pace of the breath and move in harmony with this rhythm. As you grow in confidence with the power of the breath to release and let go, begin to vocalize the out-breath, first with yawns, then sighs and groans, and perhaps long vowel sounds: 'Aah', 'Ooh', 'Eeeh' and back to 'Aaah'. Sounding the breath is an effective way to release tension, pain or discomfort.

Cat-pose explorations

To establish a comfortable base on all fours, put a folded blanket across your mat, beneath your knees for additional support. Place your hands shoulder-width apart, and slightly forward of the shoulders to give yourself more length between knees and hands. Spread the fingers very wide, so the palms are open and strong. If you experience pain in the wrists in this pose, then place a stack of yoga blocks, or even a small table or chair in front of you, at elbow height, and put the forearms on this.

All the following explorations start from a comfortable all-fours base in cat pose. Place a bolster lengthways between your knees, reaching back to your ankles, to provide support for your buttocks in the movements that swing your weight back towards the heels. Repeat each movement for as long as you are enjoying it. Your head can be held in a straight line, with the neck as a continuation of the level of the spine, or, if you prefer, you can let it hang, with the chin tucked in towards the neck. Alternate between these two options and choose the one that feels best for any given movement exploration.

1. *Rocking*

   Shift your weight forward and backwards, inhaling as it moves into the hands, and exhaling as your weight sinks back into the knees, bringing the buttocks close to the heels (or on to the bolster).

2. *Circling*

   Slowly begin to circle the whole body, spiralling out from the navel, making circles in the horizontal plane, parallel with the floor. Let the circles grow as large as feels comfortable and then spiral back down to a tiny little circle around the navel. Match the breath with the circles, using a full inhalation and exhalation to carry you round each circle. Swap directions, spiralling back the other way. For variation, use a pear shape, so that there is a narrow arc of movement across the shoulders and a wider swing across the hips.

3. *Figures of eight*

   Join up two circles: clockwise across the shoulders, and anti-clockwise from the hips. The two meet at a crossover point around the waist. Don't think about it too much though – just move in a fluid swoop across the whole body and then change direction. Let the breath flow in during one circle, and out during the other, so that each figure of eight takes one complete round of breath. At the end of these moves, experiment with some free-style wriggles, letting the body move however feels good.

4. *Basic cat*

   Keeping the lower back fairly flat, inhale and lengthen the spine, lifting the chest, neck and head up and forwards. Feel your baby hanging low into the 'hammock' made by your belly. Exhale, and round the whole back, tucking in the chin and the tailbone, and lengthening and rounding the arch in the lower back. Feel the belly muscles contracting and hugging your baby up towards your spine. Continue as long as you feel comfortable.

5. *Swooping*

   Using the exhale position from basic cat (above), sink your buttocks back towards your heels (or rest on the bolster), and keep your hands in place, with the arms stretched right out in front of you. Then, bending the elbows out to the side, keep low to the ground, inhale and swoop forwards to the level of the thumbs, before straightening the arms, and moving back to exhale and descend to the buttocks. Link these two movements to create a circling, swooping action that goes from one breath to the next with a fluid movement.

6. *Resting forwards*
Settle the buttocks on to the bolster, widen the knees slightly if necessary, ensuring there is sufficient support beneath them, then rest forwards on to a support that keeps your head and chest at the level that feels most comfortable. A birthing ball (65 or 75cm) can be the perfect height, but so too can the seat of a sofa, a chair or a beanbag. Use what's available in your home to create a comfortable nest where you can settle into this resting pose easily at the end of your cat-pose movements.

Pelvic-floor practices: breath and inner power
The forward resting pose described at the end of the previous section is the ideal base for doing pelvic-floor practices.

1. *Foundation breath with awareness*
As if you are breathing up and down the spine, on inhaling, carry the awareness up to the top of head, and exhaling, carry the awareness down to the base of the spine. Use this practice in between the others described below.

2. *Anal squeeze* (ashwini mudra)
Inhale, squeeze together the ring of muscle around the anus, and exhale, release.

3. *Urethral squeeze* (sahajoli mudra)
Inhale, squeeze together the muscles that would stop an imaginary flow of urine, and exhale, release.

4. *Vaginal squeeze and lift* (mula bandha)
Inhale, draw together the walls of the vagina, squeezing until it begins to feel as if there is a lifting upwards towards the cervix.

When practising these exercises, be sure to have the whole body relaxed except the muscles you are squeezing and releasing. Be sure too, to synchronize your breath and the muscle movement to optimize the effects of the practice. Remember it is just as important to release these muscles as it is to strengthen and squeeze them.

For more information on Uma Dinsmore-Tuli's books and website, and yoga in pregnancy, please see Resources, p. 339, and Further Reading, p. 347.

FANTASY SHOPPING

One rather inventive patient of mine told me how she did her pelvic-floor exercises. Towards the end of her pregnancy, tired or being so big that no clothes seemed to fit her any more, she dreamt of the day she could go shopping and buy herself something nice to wear. To encourage herself to do her pelvic-floor exercises she would imagine she was in the lift of her favourite department store. Her pelvic floor being the lift taking her up each floor of the store, she imagined herself stopping on the floor for shoes. She hovered there tightening her pelvic floor while she looked around the imaginary shoe department. Then, back in the lift, she went down to the dresses on the imaginary floor below. She did report that her pelvic floor made a remarkable recovery, and the shoes she bought as soon as she was able weren't bad either!

Common Conditions

Your skin

General skin conditions may actually improve while pregnant. However, you may develop skin problems you have never had before, like acne. Moles commonly get slightly bigger, which in itself is not a worry. But if they change in shape, get much bigger or raised, become itchy or bleed it is vital to get them checked out. If you have a dark rash that appears and does not fade when you press on it, it is worth having it checked.

THE SKIN IN CHINESE MEDICINE

In Chinese medicine, the skin is categorized as follows:

- Redness: Heat, normally in the Blood (see p. 59 for cooling foods you can add to your diet)
- Fluid-filled: Damp (see p. 58 for Damp-resolving foods)
- Pale, dry and flaky: Blood Deficient (see p. 57 for Blood-nourishing foods)
- Boils: Fire Poison, which is an advanced form of Heat and possibly a way of your body ridding itself of toxins (see p. 59 for Cooling foods)

Stretch marks

Stretch marks are small tears in the middle layer of the skin.

Why do they happen?

They appear when the skin's elasticity is stretched to its limits and the connective tissue tears. The marks that remain are the resulting scars which have healed.

What can you do?

Sadly, there is little that can be done to prevent stretch marks from occurring. Taking care to nourish your skin from inside and out will go some way to helping, but I do believe if you are prone to stretch marks (and this really depends on each individual's genetic make-up), there is not a great deal that will prevent them. I also think it's important not to fear your changing body shape, and while you rub oil into your bump and other areas of your body it is important to do so out of self-care. Be fascinated with your growing body and wonder in its ability to house your baby and to nourish it in the way it does.

Itchy skin

Many women experience itchy skin around the tummy area during pregnancy.

Why does it happen?

It is caused by the skin stretching, usually in the third trimester (although it can occur at any time).

What can you do?

Use plenty of moisturizer to keep the skin supple, a mild soap and make sure you are well hydrated. However, unless you are in a great deal of discomfort, I think skin conditions are best left alone until after pregnancy (except for moles, see above). If someone does present to me while pregnant I will often apply acupuncture to stop itching and to calm the mind. Skin does respond well to acupuncture and herbal medicine, but treatment is limited during pregnancy.

Note: If you itch more generally all over the body (without a rash), particularly on the soles of your feet or the palms of your hands, let your doctor or midwife know immediately, as there is a test they can do to check for a rare condition called obstetric cholestasis. This condition affects the function of the liver and may, in some cases, be dangerous to the foetus due to the build-up of bile salts in the bloodstream (which is what causes the itching). If obstetric cholestasis is diagnosed you will be carefully monitored and might be induced early. Topical aqueous cream with menthol may improve your symptoms. You may be given treatment with antihistamines or Ursodeoxycholic acid. You will probably also be given vitamin K and might want to avoid wheat and dairy products (and definitely avoid alcohol, if you are still having the odd glass of wine).

In Chinese medicine itching is a symptom of Wind and so you need to eat plenty of Blood-nourishing foods (see p. 57). If the itching is red and hot, it is also a sign of Heat and the following may help:

- ❀ Take lukewarm showers and no hot baths.
- ❀ Use aloe vera gel (keep in the fridge).
- ❀ Avoid coffee and Heating foods, like spices (see p. 58 for a full list).
- ❀ Try acupuncture – this is very effective at calming the mind and clearing Heat; patients even notice they feel cooler after treatment.[19]

MEDITATION FOR ITCHING

Lie somewhere comfortable and ask your body what it needs to feel cool and to stop itching. Does it need more Blood to go to the skin to nourish and soothe it? If so, imagine strong blood flow to the area. Or it may need a cooling light or water to bathe and soothe the itching. Spend ten minutes responding to your body's needs and feel the irritation gradually ebb away.

Colds and coughs

During pregnancy, you can be more likely to pick up coughs and colds. This is why we protect the Lung energy and also why I do tend to see conditions that stem from Cold and Damp during the third trimester.

Why does it happen?

You are often more susceptible to colds and coughs while pregnant because your immune system is likely to be slightly weaker than usual.

What can you do?

If you eat plenty of foods from the store cupboard for the third trimester (see p. 235), don't go out with wet hair (especially after swimming) and nip signs of Damp in the bud, you'll help your body to stop a sniffly cold from setting in and progressing into a condition like sinusitis (see p. 216). Comfort foods are perfect for colds, including chicken soup, of course (see recipe, p. 314), porridge and congee, a Chinese rice dish (see p. 306). Stay hydrated with herbal teas, and remember not to drink too much water with your meals.

THE IMMUNE SYSTEM IN CHINESE MEDICINE

What Western medicine would classify as a cold or the flu, in Chinese medicine we would describe as Wind invasion. Signs of Wind invasion are:

- sudden onset of cold symptoms
- dislike of the wind or cold

- neck ache
- feeling chilly
- runny nose
- sneezing.

The success or failure of a pathogen or virus to make a person unwell depends on the relative strength of the virus versus the person's defensive Qi. Here are some simple steps you can take:

- Simplify the diet and cut out refined foods and sugars.
- Cut out mucus-forming foods, including wheat, fatty foods and dairy.
- Eat soups – especially chicken (see recipe, p. 314) and cabbage.
- Drink barley water (see recipe, p. 215).
- For sore throats, gargle with salt.
- Honey and ginger are helpful – in hot drinks, for example.

Oedema

Oedema is a condition characterized by swelling and puffiness. The hands and feet are common sites for this to occur, although it can also affect the face (which normally indicates a more serious state). Often the puffiness will get worse as the day goes on or in hot weather, and will return to normal after resting or in the morning. If it does not improve, it may require medical monitoring.

Why does it happen?

Oedema is caused by fluids collecting in the body tissues. If you have oedema, your GP will look for traces of protein in the urine or an increase in blood pressure as these signs can indicate pre-eclampsia, which may cause kidney or liver damage in the mother or affect the baby's growth (see p. 221).

What can you do?

❧ Support stockings are very helpful in preventing the build-up of fluids. Make sure also that nothing you are wearing is too tight or digging in to you, such as tight shoes, tights, socks or even rings.

- ✿ Stress can lead to excessive production of anti-diuretic hormones, which results in your kidneys retaining more water, so try to eliminate all forms of stress where possible and, if you can, exercise gently, as this helps both your kidneys and the colon to eliminate more efficiently.
- ✿ Drinking fennel tea or a glass of celery juice with a dash of apple juice can help stimulate your kidneys to eliminate waste and help with water retention. Also, chamomile tea can help to reduce inflammation.
- ✿ Consider acupuncture, which can work in just one session, often relieving the body of accumulated fluids as the woman receives treatment. It really is an excellent remedy for this uncomfortable condition and I have seen it help women many times.
- ✿ Try moxibustion for oedema: St 36 for five minutes every day (see p. 112).
- ✿ Corn silk (the hairy bits found in and at the end of the corn husk) is a very good diuretic, helping to remove excess fluids from the body. Simply infuse the silk in hot water and drink like tea. This is helpful for urinary problems, high blood pressure, oedema and carpal-tunnel syndrome.
- ✿ Avoid dairy products, reduce sugar intake and consume wheat-containing foods in rotation, which means eating foods like bread, pasta, pizza, cakes and biscuits once every four days. Probiotics are also useful in supporting the gut, so that less fluid is retained.

When I was pregnant with my first daughter we lived at the top of a building, above a shop with no lift. I had cravings for watermelon and would arrive home with this huge melon and have to lug it all the way up four flights of stairs to our flat. By the end of the pregnancy it was like lugging two watermelons up those stairs but it did help with the oedema which I had a tendency towards.

Oedema in Chinese medicine

From a Chinese medicine view, there are two types of oedema: the first is Spleen Yang type and the second is Kidney Yang type and, as ever, they take slightly different approaches to treatment. Don't worry if you seem to have a mix of the two; this is not uncommon, and since both are conditions stemming from not enough Yang energy, their source is the same and there are crossovers in treatment.

Spleen Yang type

This generally affects the hands and feet and is quite mild. You may feel that you are lacking in energy and feel sluggish and tired. Your digestion may be poor and your stool loose. You may feel cold and your skin cold to the touch.

Tongue: Often chubby looking and pale.

Treatment: You need warming and you need to warm the digestive Fire so that it can transform the fluids of the body. Introduce warming foods into you diet as well as following the dietary guidelines below for both types. Don't eat overchilled or raw foods and drink water at room temperature, while taking care, as always, not to flood the system with too much water while you eat.

Kidney Yang type

The symptoms are similar to above, but this is less a digestive issue and more one of the Kidney Fire. Symptoms are likely to include backache or feeling cold in the back area.

Tongue: As with Spleen Yang, often pale and chubby.

Treatment: You need to warm the body using the moxa directions below, but you also need to rest more. Try to lie down for half an hour during the day, ideally after lunch. I know this can be hard, but it can pay significant dividends. Limit the time that you are on your feet, and spend time energizing your wrists and ankles. If you are sitting at a desk, rotate your ankles and circle your wrists.

Yoga for swollen ankles/wrists/ carpal-tunnel syndrome

Yoga tip: breathe and move to keep the energy flowing freely.

Practice: energy block release for the feet and hands

If the feet, wrists and ankles swell during pregnancy they can become very tender and stiff. A combination of mindful yoga breath and movement can restore mobility and encourage proper drainage of the accumulating fluid. These practices only work, however, if the movements are done very slowly, and are always accompanied with a full breath and mindful attention. Repeat each action up to eleven times.

To relieve stiffness and swelling in the ankles and feet, sit with your legs out straight, a little wider than your mat. If this position aggravates lower-back pain, sit on a cushion or the edge of a folded blanket. You can lean back on to your arms, placing your hands behind you, a little wider than your hips. Use *ujayii* breath (see p. 196) and, as you inhale, open up as much space as possible between all the toes on both feet, stretching them wide. Exhale, curl the toes under and squeeze tight closed. Repeat up to eleven times.

Take the same action into the ankles: inhale, and push into the heels, straightening the legs and moving the toes back towards the hips. Exhale, point the toes to the ground. Repeat the same number of times as for the toe squeezes.

With all the toes pointing straight up, and legs straight, inhale, and as you do so, draw the outer sides of the feet back towards your hips. Exhaling, draw the outside edges of the foot in towards the centre, feeling the strength in the inner arch of the foot. Repeat the same number of times as previous exercises.

Circle the feet very slowly in opposite directions, breathing in as your toes move away from you, and out as they move towards you. Do the same number of repetitions in each direction.

If wrists are swollen or movement is painful, you can ease mobility by using the same sequence for the hands, holding out your arms at slightly below shoulder height, and breathing into the rhythmic movement of the fingers, hands and wrists, in the same pattern as described above for the feet and ankles.

For a full programme of joint- and energy-freeing poses to do against the wall during pregnancy, see Uma Dinsmore-Tuli's books and website.

REFLEXOLOGY FOR FLUID RETENTION

A qualified maternity reflexologist should be able to help reduce the swelling and discomfort in front of your very eyes, although if you aren't lucky enough to be able to visit one, there are some areas you can work on yourself.

Reflex areas

The wrist/ankle: a nice easy tip to help swollen ankles is to work on your own cross reflex – the wrist (cross reflexes are anatomical parts of the body, which are energetically connected to another part of the body). Use a wringing technique around the whole of the wrist area to reduce swelling within the ankles – it's a bit like giving yourself a Chinese burn with one hand, but obviously don't go in too hard!

Lymphatics: to help aid drainage, make little downward pinching movements between each finger on the hand (both sides of the finger simultaneously) to halfway down, then drag back up between the fingers, with a quick sharp movement.

BARLEY WATER

Barley water is an excellent remedy for removing dampness from the body. The addition of ginger makes it warming in nature, so it will have the added benefit of tonifying Yang and supporting the digestion.

Note: For Damp Heat conditions, omit the ginger in this recipe.

Makes just under 1.5 litres (2½ pints)

150g (5½oz) pearl barley

zest and juice of 2 lemons

1 tablespoon finely grated fresh ginger

4 tablespoons honey

1. Rinse the barley in a sieve under the tap, until the water runs clear. Put in a saucepan with the lemon zest, ginger and 1.5 litres (2½ pints) of water.

2. Bring the mixture to the boil, then simmer for 10 minutes.
3. Strain the liquid, then stir in the honey, 1 tablespoon at a time, to dissolve in the liquid. Stir in the lemon juice, then set aside to cool. Store in the refrigerator. Except on the warmest days, bring to room temperature before serving.

LYMPHATIC DRAINAGE AND PREGNANCY

The lymphatic system is a vast network of capillaries and nodes that removes and destroys the toxic substances, transports the nutrients such as vitamins, minerals and hormones throughout the body and eliminates excess fluid from the tissues.

Manual Lymphatic Drainage (MLD) is a very gentle, subtle, repetitive form of massage, based on pumping and scooping movements which encourage fluids to flow more freely around the body. This renews, nourishes, strengthens and regenerates the cells, removes waste products and relaxes the nervous system. It is an excellent treatment for tired and heavy legs.

During pregnancy, the body retains more fluid than at other times. As the foetus starts to grow, it puts pressure on the lymphatic nodes and capillaries in the pelvis and the abdomen and inguinal areas; the flow of the fluid from the lower extremities slows down and the legs become heavier, especially around the knees and ankles. Sometimes the legs become so heavy that it may cause discomfort or even pain.

The movements of MLD are extremely gentle and based purely on touch, so it is a therapy that can be applied throughout pregnancy.

Sinusitis

I have found sinusitis to be quite common in my pregnant patients. There is not a distinct pattern of symptoms; often, it is a progression from a cold to a more stubborn condition where the Phlegm is hard to shift and pain persists in the sinus area.

Why does it happen?

There are a couple of possibilities as to why sinusitis affects women during pregnancy.

Here in the UK, we live in a damp climate and are therefore far more prone to Damp problems which can progress into conditions characterized by Phlegm. One of my acupuncture colleagues from Australia complains that whenever she arrives at Heathrow, she immediately lays down a layer of cellulite (Damp) which stays firmly on her thighs until she leaves.

A second possibility is that pregnant women tend to generate Dampness more easily, and it's also harder to shift in a pregnant woman.

What can you do?

All in all, I find this a stubborn condition to treat. However, there are some things that you can do to help manage sinusitis and some of the self-help suggestions I give here are really effective.

Sinusitis often follows on from a cold, so keeping the immune system strong will help prevent its onset. It is also worth keeping in mind that Phlegm is generated through the digestive system, so taking care of your digestive functions and being good to your Spleen (see p. 178) will help prevent Phlegm from generating in the first place.

Inhalations can be helpful and eucalyptus is safe as an essential oil in small doses. Use two drops of the oil on a tissue or add to a bowl of hot water to use as a steam inhalation with a towel over your head.

Damp Heat type

Blocked up-nose with lost sense of smell and pain in the face. There may be yellow discharge or no discharge at all, as the Phlegm is so deeply set.

Tongue: Swollen and coated, generally with a yellow coating.

Treatment: Avoid too many Phlegm-forming foods like dairy, peanuts, concentrated juices such as orange and tomato, sugar and fatty foods. Many women actually increase their dairy intake during pregnancy in the belief that they need increased calcium and this has the knock-on effect of increasing Dampness and Phlegm in their system. There are other very good sources of calcium, such as sesame seeds and leafy green vegetables; a dish I find helpful is leafy greens lightly steamed in a wok with some soy sauce and a sprinkling of sesame seeds.

Foods to clear Phlegm include almonds, apple peel, button mush-rooms, garlic, grapefruit, lemon peel, liquorice, marjoram, mustard seeds, olives, onions, orange peel, pears, peppers, peppermint, seaweed, shiitake mushrooms, thyme, walnuts and watercress.

SALT NOSE WASH FOR SINUS PROBLEMS

If you've never tried using a neti pot, it does take a bit of getting used to, but after a short period of adjustment, you will soon be looking forward to incorporating it into your daily routine – it will become second nature, like cleaning your teeth and washing your face.

In this ancient Ayurvedic practice, a pot is filled with lukewarm saltwater which is then poured through each nostril. Do this carefully, tilting your head at the right angle, to allow the water to flow through the other nostril, clearing away dust, dirt and pollen, and flushing your tear ducts.

For allergy sufferers and those with sinus problems, it is a natural solu-tion that can, eventually, replace medication. And for those of you who just want to rid yourselves of the pollutants of city life, it's a useful practice to add into your daily routine, giving you a clear head.

A couple of tips when getting used to your neti pot:

- Pay attention to the amount of salt you use, and adjust according to your level of comfort.
- The temperature of the water is key – use a little boiling water to dissolve the salt crystals and then add cold water, until it is the same temperature as your skin.

Reflexology for sinusitis

Reflexology can be very effective in helping with the pain associated with sinusitis; it can drain the sinuses and help strengthen the area to prevent repeat sinusitis attacks.

Reflex areas to treat

Sinus areas: All of the fingers represent the sinus area, so using the 'caterpil-lar' technique (see p. 335), work from either the tip down to the base of each finger or, alternatively, from the base to the tip. If there is significant pain, squeezing the fingers can also help to relieve symptoms very quickly.

Repeat a few times on each finger, or until symptoms disappear.

Carpal-tunnel syndrome

Carpal-tunnel syndrome is pain in the hand caused by an increase of fluid in the wrist joint pressing on the nerve.

Why does it happen?

This is caused by water retention or congestion in your pregnancy. The nerve becomes compressed in a very tight space and gives you pins and needles. You will probably find it is worse at night, especially if you curl your wrists up while sleeping. This can be avoided by wearing a wrist brace before going to bed.

What can you do?

There are a number of things you can try which might help ease discomfort:

- ❀ Try this simple 'wrist-wringing' technique. Clasp one wrist with your other hand and massage it with a circular movement. This will ease congestion and encourage fluid movement.
- ❀ Avoid movements that are painful, and exercise your hands and arms gently to stretch them.
- ❀ Try hanging your hands over the edge of your bed during the night. If you wake up with pain, try shaking your hands until the pain or numbness goes away.
- ❀ Some women find it useful to place their hands in ice-cold water or hold a bag of frozen peas against the painful area of their wrists.
- ❀ Gently exercising your fingers and wrists can help to move the excess fluid back into your circulation, and keeping your hands raised as much as possible may also be beneficial.
- ❀ Carpal-tunnel reflex: symptoms may be eased by working across the bracelet of the wrist (inside only) using the 'caterpillar' technique (see p. 335). If you can, after each step, push in and circle before moving on. Repeat for sixty seconds.

Carpal-tunnel syndrome in Chinese medicine

In Chinese medicine, too much Dampness accumulating locally can block the flow of Qi in the channels and tissues. This leads to a feeling of heaviness, numbness and aching. An accumulation of fluid in an upper-body area like the wrists is seen as a reflection of a weakness of the Lungs to transform fluids. The following can be helpful:

❀ Introduce foods to remove Damp like adzuki beans, garlic and spring greens.
❀ Avoid Dampening foods like wheat, orange juice and dairy products.
❀ Don't eat late at night.
❀ Acupuncture has been shown to be effective.[20, 21]

Small for dates

I see an increasing number of women who are told their babies are small for dates. Your baby's growth will be assessed by the midwife by measuring the symphyseal-fundal height (the distance from your pubic bone to the top of the uterus). This is measured in centimetres and, conveniently, the number of centimetres approximately matches the number of weeks of your pregnancy (so for example, at twenty-eight weeks the symphyseal-fundal height should measure about 28cm). If the measurement is significantly smaller than expected, the midwife or obstetrician may arrange an ultrasound scan to assess growth and well-being.

Small babies may be termed either 'small for gestational age' or 'growth restricted'.

Why does it happen?

Small-for-gestational-age babies are usually small due to constitutional factors (such as the mother's size, family history or ethnicity). These babies are small, but show normal growth, and they are usually delivered at term. In contrast, growth-restricted babies (who show intrauterine growth restriction – IUGR) are small due to placental insufficiency. Chronic illness or illness during pregnancy can be a cause of growth restriction, as can smoking in pregnancy. Growth-restricted babies usually have reduced growth velocity and may have to be delivered early. In such cases, both mother and baby will be monitored closely by a midwife or obstetrician. If the baby shows signs of distress, the obstetrician may decide the best course of action is to deliver early by Caesarean section (see p. 277). Or, if the pregnancy goes to term and the baby is still considered very small, the advice might be to have the baby in a hospital with a special-care baby unit. Growth restriction may also be associated with pre-eclampsia.

What can you do?

Following the healthy-living advice in this and other books can make a real difference, especially good diet, plenty of rest and relaxation. When I first started to see women who were being diagnosed with small-for-dates babies, there was very little in my Chinese medicine books to help me. I observed that most of these women were working long hours and tended to be Blood Deficient. Helping to nourish the mother's Blood may increase the blood flow available to the baby and increase its growth. I have seen an improvement many times simply by teaching the mother to moxa St 36 every day. Here are some suggestions you could try, if your obstetrician or midwife is happy for you to do so:

- ❀ Moxa on St 36 for ten days (see diagram on p. 112) is an excellent treatment when given in conjunction with your obstetrician's care.
- ❀ Rest is vital – consider going on maternity leave earlier than you'd intended.
- ❀ Increase nourishing foods like chicken soup (see recipe, p. 314), leafy greens, sweet potatoes, casseroles, eggs, rice, oats, ginger, rosemary, dates, kidney beans, porridge with cinnamon, cardamom and berries or dates and apricots.
- ❀ Avoid Cold and raw foods.

Hypertension/ pre-eclampsia

Your blood pressure will be measured regularly during your pregnancy. Blood pressure usually falls in the first trimester and increases gradually towards pre-pregnancy levels during the second and third trimesters. A significant rise in blood pressure, however, may be a concern. For some women it may be associated with protein in the urine and swelling – a condition called pre-eclampsia. It's important to keep up with your antenatal visits as they will routinely include tests to pick it up early and manage with treatment. Early symptoms might include sudden weight gain, excessive swelling in your fingers, wrists and ankles and a drop in the amount of urine you are passing. For some women, however, there are no early signs.

Why does it happen?

Pre-eclampsia is a result of abnormal, early placental development. Treated early, it can be controlled and pose no long-term health threats to you or your baby. If not picked up, however, it may affect your baby's growth, and also puts strain on your kidneys, heart and nervous system, sometimes causing severe damage to blood vessels. In pre-eclampsia, there is thought to be a high level of inflammation in the body. A question that science is asking is: if the maternal inflammatory response can be dampened down, could pre-eclampsia rates be reduced?[22] Interestingly, very few of my pregnant patients develop pre-eclampsia, which has led me to question if acupuncture is reducing inflammation and thereby preventing the condition.

Severe pre-eclampsia is rare and the symptoms tend to occur later in pregnancy, or occasionally after birth. They include:

- ❀ headaches
- ❀ stomach aches
- ❀ blurred or altered vision
- ❀ feeling very unwell
- ❀ confusion and disorientation
- ❀ shortness of breath.

Treating pre-eclampsia

When picked up in the early stages, pre-eclampsia may be controlled with rest and treatment, if necessary, to lower the blood pressure (antihypertensives). Hospital admission for close monitoring may be necessary if you have both hypertension and protein in the urine. And once back at home, you'll need to keep a close eye out for any returning symptoms. Reducing the salt in your diet is worthwhile and making sure you eat a healthy diet.

In later pregnancy, your obstetrician may decide, when considering all the factors of your pregnancy, to either induce labour or deliver the baby by Caesarean section, if necessary.

HIGH BLOOD PRESSURE IN CHINESE MEDICINE – LEARNING TO BE A FREE-AND-EASY WANDERER

In Chinese medicine, the Liver is associated with anger and hostility, so it is important to keep the Liver happy and free-flowing in order to keep the blood pressure low. Learning to keep your cool and not to get too heated about things is important for Liver health. Equally, deeply held resentments and hostility can put pressure on the Liver. It's a bit like a pressure cooker effect: the excess energy rises to the top of the body as the pressure builds.

Learning to deal with your anger and practising forgiveness are very important in managing blood pressure. This long-held Chinese medicine idea is beginning to be backed up by modern research.[23] Our Liver energy is said to be healthy when we have a strong vision of where our life is going and the ability to carry out what is in our mind's eye. When this is thwarted, we become frustrated and the pressure builds internally. Also, frequent positive support from a partner has been shown to result in higher levels of oxytocin (see p. 265) and sustained lower blood pressure.[24] Yoga, tai qi, acupuncture and reflexology are all useful, but changing the way we approach life is vital.

Liver-cleansing Dandelion, Chicory and Coriander Salad

Dandelion is an extremely good tonic for draining excess Damp from the body, as is chicory. Coriander is a Qi mover, if you are feeling a little Stagnant in the digestive department.

Makes 4 side salads

3 medium chicory heads (also known as Belgian endive)
about 25 young dandelion leaves
1 bunch fresh coriander
¼–½ teaspoon sea salt
½ large juicy lemon, or 1 smaller lemon
2½ tablespoons extra-virgin olive oil

1. Thinly slice the chicory crosswise and separate the half-rings as you put them into a salad bowl.
2. Rinse the dandelion leaves and dry in a salad spinner. Using kitchen scissors, chop the leaves into small pieces until you have about three handfuls and add to the bowl. You can use some of the dandelion stalks, but the taste becomes increasingly bitter as the stalk gets bigger, so add according to your taste.
3. Rinse and dry the coriander. Again, using kitchen scissors, chop the leaves off the stalks until you have about two handfuls and add to the bowl.
4. Add salt to taste (start sparingly and add more when the salad is dressed).
5. Squeeze the lemon over the bowl, using your other hand to catch and discard the pips. Using both hands, lightly mix the greens, making sure the salt and lemon are well dispersed. Add the olive oil and mix together.

Vaginal discharge and itching

It is fairly common for women to experience an increase in vaginal secretions when pregnant, particularly in the last few months. The question of what constitutes 'normal' will to some extent depend on the individual. Broadly speaking, a discharge that is milky (or watery) white and does not have an odour would be considered normal. However, a discharge that is yellow or green and has an odour, and/or itching or inflammation of the vagina may indicate infection and needs medical attention.

Why does it happen?

The causes for infection can be sexually transmitted disease, often passed back and forth between partners (in which case, both partners should be treated). Bacteria such as gardnerella can also lead to bacterial vaginosis.

In Chinese medicine terms, there are two slight variations of this condition, as follows:

Dampness

Arising from poor digestion. Tiredness with vaginal discharge (without much smell), vaginal itching and a loose stool.

Tongue: Pale, with a white coat.

Treatment: Since this manifestation has its roots in digestive weakness, the diet is a good place to start. Make sure that you keep your diet simple and avoid all Damp-forming foods, such as sugar, chocolate, orange juice, bread, yeast, bananas, dairy products and pork. Foods to include are adzuki beans, barley, celery, green tea, lemon, coriander, mackerel, marjoram, parsley, onions, pumpkin and rye.

Acupressure point: St 36.

Dampness combined with Heat (affecting the Liver channel)

The Liver channel runs up the inside of the leg and circles the genitals in both men and women, so it is often involved in problems associated with that area. You may remember that the Liver is easily affected by emotional issues, such as frustration and anger, so it is important to keep this in mind, I will suggest ways to help if you think this is you.

The itching is intense and there may be a general swelling and strong discharge. You feel emotionally irritable and 'hot and bothered' – you may notice that your body temperature is running a bit high and generally feel your body is hot and moist to the touch (but not always).

Tongue: Red, yellow coat (especially at the back).

Treatment: You too need to clean up the diet by avoiding both Heat- and Damp-forming foods (see p. 31); dairy, concentrated juices, absolutely no alcohol (for those who are having the odd one) and sugar.
Acupressure point: Liv 3 (see p. 112).

Breech

Your baby will hopefully be settled head down in the pelvis by between weeks 34 and 36. Your midwife will palpate your belly (feel with her hands) to check the position of your baby and can also show you how to recognize the various bumps and kicks. Although many babies will move into the correct position during week 35 or 36 (even later sometimes), I feel it is worth following the ten-day moxibustion cycle (see below) from week 34, as some research suggests more babies will turn with this treatment than without.[25] Further-more, it is a very simple and inexpensive technique that could prevent the need for medical intervention.

Unfortunately, although many medical practitioners now promote the use of moxibustion, they normally do so once it is too late to turn the baby. Typically, at around week 39, I will get a call from a patient saying her midwife has suggested she tries acupuncture and moxibustion. With the best will in the world, there is very little room left for turning by this stage. My experi-ence is that it does work very well, but rather than being a last resort, it is much more effective as a first-line non-invasive intervention in babies that are breech from thirty-four weeks. Having said that, I have had babies turn with moxibustion as late as week 39, especially when the woman has already had a baby, but it's not the norm.

Breech, or indeed any malposition of a baby, is viewed in terms of insuffi-ciency of Yang energy. Birth requires a great deal of Yang activity, and if there has been either Qi Stagnation or Deficiency building up over the pregnancy then there will not be sufficient Yang a) to hold the baby in the correct posi-tion and b) to sustain the mother's Yang energy through the birth process. The purpose of the ten-day moxibustion treatment is to increase Yang activ-ity in the uterus to encourage the baby to turn.

Ten-day moxibustion treatment cycle

Leading obstetric acupuncturist Debra Betts outlines the following treatment in her book *The Essential Guide to Acupuncture in Pregnancy and Childbirth*. For additional guidelines on how to light and extinguish the moxa, see p. 333.

❀ Moxibustion (moxa) is used on the acupuncture/ acupressure point Bl 67 for ten days.

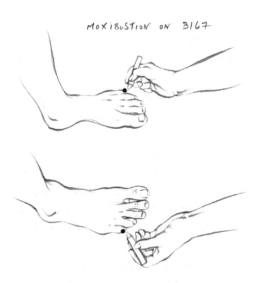

MOXIBUSTION ON Bl67

Bl67 IS USED WITH MOXA AS SHOWN TO TURN BREECH BABIES; IT CAN ALSO BE USED IN LABOUR WITH EAR-PRESS SEEDS TO ENCOURAGE A POSTERIOR BABY INTO A BETTER POSITION

❀ It is best for the woman's partner to do this treatment since the point is on the little toe.
❀ Sit in a comfortable position with legs extended out in front of you.
❀ Your partner can use two moxa sticks simultaneously, holding them over each point on the little toe on each foot.

- ❀ The sticks will need to be a thumb-width away from the skin to prevent overheating.
- ❀ Sticks should be held in position until the point becomes hot, then removed briefly before returning them to the point.
- ❀ Continue this for twenty minutes.
- ❀ Do this every day for ten days.
- ❀ Treatment needs to be continued for the full ten days even if/ when the baby turns. However, at this point you may halve the amount of time to ten minutes.

Note: You *should not* use this treatment if you have had a previous breech baby or if you have high blood pressure. Check with your healthcare provider.

What is interesting about this treatment is that as the Yang increases in the uterus, you will notice more activity from your baby. Typically, halfway through the course, the baby's activity peaks. It is important to accept that not all babies will turn and, indeed, some women's uterus shape does not allow the baby to turn easily into the head-down position. In some cases, when the baby has not turned and there is time, I might suggest trying the ten-day treatment again. I have seen this work in women who have previously had successful vaginal deliveries or where we know the baby is not breech due to uterus shape.

However, some women get to the point where they are happy to let things be. Coming to terms with a breech baby and, in some cases, letting go of the idea of a vaginal delivery can be hard though, and I think it is important to resolve these disappointments and to spend time exploring your feelings around them. Of course, many women are very pragmatic and can easily move into a place where they can accept the birth, however it is, just so long as both they and their babies are safe.

EAR-PRESS SEEDS

These are minute seeds, or grains, with a plaster on them that can be placed on Bl 67 (see diagram, p. 227) during labour. I normally suggest these in the case of babies who have been in the posterior position, even if they turn back. Treatment may not change the position of the baby, but it usually eases backache.

- During labour ask your partner or midwife to apply the seed over Bl 67 on both toes.
- Place a plaster around the ear-press seed to keep it in place.
- Replace as needed.
- Your partner can also apply pressure to points Bl 60 and SP 6 (see p. 269, for acupressure during labour).

Induction

The exact expected due date of a baby has become something of an unhealthy preoccupation for the modern pregnant woman. Pregnancy is measured in weeks and often monitored on a day-to-day basis as the date looms nearer. This creates a great deal of tension and frustration when the baby does not arrive exactly 'on time'. Although statistics show that the optimal time for delivery is between thirty-eight and forty weeks, my feeling has always been that we need to weigh up the perceived dangers of letting women go over their due date (often hospitals will induce from forty-one weeks), with the complications that can ensue following an induction. Probably the best solution is to treat each case individually.

Unfortunately, the over-focus on due date and the fact that women are warned from a very early stage about not going more than two weeks over this date has resulted in an increase in anxiety for the woman, especially during the last few days of pregnancy when peace should be the order of the day. Some first-time mothers believe that they will be unable to go into labour without an induction, and that this will automatically mean that they will have a more difficult labour. It is a great shame that so many women spend the last few weeks of their pregnancy obsessing about whether or not they will go into labour 'on time' and this becomes the preoccupation of what should be a very special time. From a Chinese medicine viewpoint, this frustration causes the Liver energy to stagnate, which, ironically, could result in delaying labour. In the wild, an animal would never go into labour if it felt it was not safe to do so. It is the same for humans; we need to feel relaxed and secure.

As an acupuncturist, I am called upon more and more frequently to help women 'go into labour'. I do not think that acupuncture will make a woman go into labour if the physiological processes that initiate it are not ready and in process. I think that acupuncture is excellent as a preparation for labour, but there are no studies to show that inducing a labour with acupuncture is any more or less 'natural' than a medical induction. My aim is always to help make women feel calm, safe, secure and never hurried. In my clinic I offer two approaches.

The first is pre-birth acupuncture and consists of three to four treatments given in the last trimester, leading up to labour to help prepare the woman. The aim here is to build her Qi and Blood and prepare the cervix.

The second approach is for women who are already booked in for a medical induction. This treatment is given twenty-four hours prior to the induction procedure. My experience and the feedback I have received from obstetricians who refer patients for this treatment is that the induction process is often more effective and progresses more easily when the woman has had acupuncture as an adjunct treatment.

Acupressure

Where acupuncture is not available, and you know you are to be induced on a certain day, it is well worth trying acupressure in the days before. Points LI 4, Sp 6 and Bl 32 are the ones to use (see Acupressure for labour, p. 269). Use the points for three to five minutes, two hours apart.

Note: if the amniotic fluid (your waters) are discoloured – usually brown or green – let your midwife know straight away; they will need to get labour started more quickly.

Reflexology

If you're overdue, or worried about being overdue, bear in mind that just like acupuncture, reflexology can't be used as a quick-fix last resort before a medical induction; a one-off treatment won't generally be enough. The body has to have time to adapt, so I would urge all pregnant women to see a reflexologist at least six to eight weeks before their due date. There are a couple of techniques you can help yourself with though (after thirty-seven weeks only):

Reflex areas to treat
Pituitary reflex
Using the 'tornado' technique (see p. 335), you can work your own pituitary reflex (middle of each thumb) to stimulate the hormone oxytocin, which will help bring on a natural birth – the best way to do this is to use the knuckle of your index finger to push in and rotate on each opposite thumb for sixty seconds each. Repeat and revisit as often as you can (This can also be used after birth to help with milk production, rebalancing hormones and helping to overcome postnatal depression.)

Uterus and ovaries
For the uterus reflex, turn your hand facing downwards. At the base of the wrist, below the thumb, find the small indentation and stimulate for thirty to sixty seconds using the 'tornado' technique (see p. 335)

The ovaries are directly opposite, on the other side of the wrist, in the indentation underneath the little finger. (A tip for finding these spots easily is to wave gently side to side, as if you're the Queen! Place your fingers on the outside of your wrists and the indentations will become very clear.) Repeat three times.

REASONS FOR INDUCTION

There are several reasons why a decision may be taken to induce.

Prolonged pregnancy

If pregnancy goes into the forty-second week, it is considered a prolonged pregnancy and there is a risk that the placenta will then start to deteriorate, affecting the supply of oxygen and nutrients to the baby. Remember that the due date is estimated, it is not set in stone, and only about 5 per cent of women go into labour on this date. Your midwife or obstetrician should ask you about your cycle pre-pregnancy. If you had a slightly longer cycle – more than twenty-eight days – then your natural due date might well be later than that in your notes.

Waters break, but labour doesn't start

If your waters break, but labour doesn't spontaneously start within twenty-four hours, your healthcare team may discuss induction with you to avoid the risk of infection. However, this is an arbitrary time limit and if you want to push to leave it a bit longer, do talk to your midwife.

The baby isn't thriving

In some pregnancies, the placenta begins to deteriorate before the due date and the foetus may fail to continue to thrive. Induction will then be discussed, as it may be healthier for your baby to be born sooner.

Vaginal bleeding in late pregnancy

Again, vaginal bleeding may indicate that the placenta is no longer working efficiently and may be coming away from the uterine wall. Any vaginal bleeding will be investigated thoroughly by your obstetrician and the option to induce might be considered the best course of action.

Pre-existing conditions or illness

If you have any conditions that may affect your own safety and that of your baby – for example, heart disease, diabetes or if you have developed high blood pressure or pre-eclampsia during pregnancy – you may be induced early.

What happens during induction?

Before induction is considered your midwife should offer you a membrane sweep to help you go into labour. This is a vaginal examination to assess the cervix and its favourability. Cervical assessment is useful to assess the chances that you'll go into labour spontaneously. The midwife will place a finger into the cervix and make a sweeping movement to separate the membranes that surround the baby, often stimulating labour. A sweep has no risk to the baby, but may cause a small amount of vaginal bleeding or discomfort and reduces the risk of a formal (medical) induction. It can be repeated as necessary.

To induce, prostaglandins, which act like the body's natural hormones to trigger labour, will be inserted into your vagina in gel, tablet or pessary form in the morning. If given as a tablet or gel, contractions will ideally start around six hours later, or twenty-four hours later with a pessary. If you don't go into labour, your midwife will talk you through the option of another dose of prostaglandins, or the option of Caesarean section (see p. 276) may be discussed, especially if your baby is showing any signs of distress.

Amniotomy is a method of induction where your waters are artificially broken. It is more likely to be offered to help speed up a very slow labour. A small plastic hooked instrument is used to puncture the membrane containing the amniotic fluid. The results are often unpredictable and an amniotomy may be used in combination with a syntocinon drip – this uses a concentrated synthetic form of oxytocin, a hormone which, in labour, triggers contractions. Syntocinon can induce very strong contractions very quickly, however, which means not being able to build up gradually. Hence an epidural often goes hand in hand with syntocinon.

The domino effect of induction in terms of pain relief and medical intervention means that induction is something you need to be fully informed about. You need to feel confident that it is the right course of action for you and your baby, which it definitely can be in some cases. If, however, it's a matter of being a few days over your due date, do ask questions to make sure.

WHAT YOU CAN TRY TO GET THINGS GOING

If you are keen to get things going, try the following:

- By keeping moving, you may help your baby's head to increase the pressure on your cervix, but don't overdo it as you need to be storing up your energy at this time.
- Sex and specifically orgasm is thought to be a trigger for contractions in some women.
- Visualizing your baby's position and the journey moving down the birth canal is a good preparation exercise in any case, and might just help to get things moving if it's the right time.

Is the Fuel Good?

Most of your baby's organs are developed by about halfway through pregnancy, but your baby's brain has a real growth spurt during the third trimester. Getting enough calories, protein and omega-3 fatty acids in your diet is, therefore, important in the last few months of pregnancy. The majority of pregnant women are advised to increase their calorie intake by about five hundred during the third trimester, as it is a time of such significant growth for your baby, but your doctor or midwife will give you more individual advice depending on your pregnancy up to this point.

While it's essential to make sure you get adequate calories, it's also good to eat little and often through the day, rather than eat big meals, as heartburn and indigestion can be common throughout pregnancy and especially during the third trimester. If you include plenty of complex carbohydrates in your diet, you will also help to keep fatigue at bay as energy releases slowly through the day. Avoiding too many fatty or rich foods will also help prevent heartburn, and including foods high in fibre and hydration will help ease constipation.

Eating well during your pregnancy also has beneficial effects in the long term, both for you and your bump. Good nutrition is part of the important preparation for both labour and early motherhood: a healthy diet has been linked with helping women carry to term and it also builds up your energy and endurance reserves for labour. Postpartum, you will need these reserves to nurture your body's recovery and also care for your newborn baby. And continuing your healthy diet habits beyond pregnancy will contribute to your own general health and well-being throughout life.

Many of the common conditions I see during the third trimester tend to be of a Damp disposition, so I also look to build Lung Qi and avoid too many Damp- or Phlegm-inducing foods during this time. The focus continues to be on nourishing the Blood and preparing the body, and your kitchen cupboards, for becoming a mum.

Store cupboard for the third trimester

- ❀ Grains: barley, rice
- ❀ Vegetables: asparagus, celery, leafy greens, fennel, onions, olives, pumpkin, watercress, button mushrooms, shiitake mushrooms, seaweed
- ❀ Fruit: grapefruit, lemons, pears, plums
- ❀ Beans: adzuki, kidney, mung
- ❀ Fish: sardines, mackerel (limit to two portions a week)
- ❀ Nuts and seeds: almonds, chestnuts, walnuts; sunflower, pumpkin, white and black sesame seeds
- ❀ Aromatic herbs and spices: basil, cardamom, coriander, garlic, liquorice, marjoram, mustard seeds, pepper, peppermint, thyme

Soothing Fennel and Chestnut Soup

A creamy and filling soup to nourish all types. I am a big fan of chestnuts, as they are not only delicious and remind me of Christmas, but they are extremely good for the digestion, as is fennel.

Serves 4–6

450g (1lb) chestnuts
olive oil
1 medium onion, peeled and chopped into quarters

3 large garlic cloves, peeled
2 or 3 celery stalks with leaves, roughly chopped
1 fennel bulb with fronds, roughly sliced (use the fronds for the garnish)
1 bay leaf
sea salt and pepper, to taste
1 litre (1¾ pints) water or chicken stock
30g (1oz) butter

1. Preheat the oven to 220°C/425°F/gas mark 7.
2. Rinse the chestnuts and carefully score the sides with a sharp paring knife, making an X or a V shape. Place the chestnuts on a baking tray, scored side up, and roast in the preheated oven for 20 minutes (see if they're done by inserting the knife into the middle – it should be tender). Remove from the oven and set aside to cool. Reduce the oven temperature to 190°C/375°F/gas mark 5.
3. Pour a couple of glugs of olive oil into a glass or ceramic baking dish and cover with the onion, garlic, celery, fennel and bay leaf. Season with sea salt and add a quarter of the water or stock. Cook in the oven for about 30 minutes; until the vegetables are translucent and soft, but not charred. While they're cooking, peel the chestnuts, removing as much of the inner skin as possible and chop into quarters or smaller.
4. Remove the vegetables from the oven and put in a large saucepan with a couple more glugs of olive oil, the remainder of the stock or water, the butter and the chestnuts (removing the bay leaf). Bring to the boil, then simmer for 15 minutes with the lid on.
5. Allow to cool, then using a food processor or high-powered blender, whizz to a smooth, creamy consistency in small batches. Serve with crusty bread and butter and a salad for lunch, or in little bowls as a starter.

Pear Crisp with Almonds and Walnuts

Of all the fruits, pears are the most Phlegm-clearing, and almonds and walnuts do the same job. This makes a great breakfast as well as a hearty, but healthy, pud!

Serves 6

4 pears, ripe but firm
30ml (1fl oz) lemon juice
1 vanilla pod (optional)
2–4 tablespoons agave syrup, or 4–6 tablespoons brown sugar
    (depending on desired sweetness)
100ml (3½fl oz) water
90g (3oz) walnuts
200g (7oz) ground almonds
½ teaspoon salt
30g (1oz) butter, chilled (plus a little more for baking)

1. Preheat the oven to 220°C/425°F/gas mark 7.
2. Core, peel and slice the pears. Halve the vanilla pod lengthways and scrape out the seeds.
3. In a large pan, over medium–high heat, melt 15g (½oz) butter, then add the pears and vanilla seeds. Sauté for a minute or two, then add 1–2 tablespoons agave or 2–3 tablespoons sugar, followed by half the water. Sauté for a few minutes more; the pears should caramelize a bit, and then add the rest of the water.
4. When the pears are a pale golden brown and the liquid is syrupy, squeeze over the lemon juice, remove from the heat and set aside.
5. Crush the walnuts gently with a rolling pin – it's helpful to keep them in a bag as you do this – you don't want powder, but a nice variety of different-sized pieces.
6. Add the ground almonds to a mixing bowl with the salt and stir.
7. Cut half the butter into tiny pieces and add to the ground almonds. Add 1–2 tablespoons agave or 2–3 tablespoons sugar to the almonds and

butter, and mix it together with your hands, lightly crumbling it between your fingers until it resembles fine breadcrumbs. Stir in the walnuts.

8. Place the pear mixture in a 20cm square (8 x 8in), or a 23cm (9in) diameter round baking dish and add the almond and walnut mixture, covering evenly and pressing it around the edges with your fingers. Dot the top with little slivers of the remaining butter. Bake for 15–18 minutes, until the top is brown and the pear mixture is bubbling. Remove from the oven and leave to cool for 20 minutes before serving.

Heartburn/acid reflux

Heartburn is a painful burning sensation, often around your breastbone and up to your lower throat.

Why does it happen?

Heartburn is caused by acid from the stomach being brought up into the oesophagus. This is thought to be a result of pregnancy hormones and, later in pregnancy, your baby slowing digestion and elimination. In Chinese medicine, heartburn is congestion, Stagnation or Heat in the digestion.

What can you do?

It is a good idea to keep a diary to help you identify triggers in your lifestyle and diet that may be causing the heartburn – then certain foods can be avoided to minimize symptoms. Identifying the source of 'the Fire', as we say in Chinese medicine, is to find the solution.

Here are a few suggestions that might help:

- ❀ Breathing deep and slow can ease heartburn by helping to keep the acid reflux to a minimum, optimizing fluid mechanics.
- ❀ Don't lie down too soon after eating, as it's much easier for the acid to go into reverse, up into your oesophagus this way.
- ❀ Sleeping propped up with many pillows can provide relief.
- ❀ A simple salad of pineapple and papaya with lemon juice and mint will help to ease heartburn and indigestion.

- ✿ Grated white radish with a small dash of soy sauce works a treat.
- ✿ Reduce fatty foods; and if you have a strong digestion, raw foods can be helpful here – in particular, bitter salad leaves.
- ✿ Mung bean soup or cabbage soup are both excellent.
- ✿ Sip peppermint tea.
- ✿ Avoid fizzy drinks and orange juice.

Reflexology for heartburn

Reflexology helps to return the healing energy to the whole stomach area and to encourage normal functioning.

Reflex areas to treat

Stomach: Massaging the entire web area between the thumb and forefinger with a 'caterpillar' technique (see p. 335). Continue until you've covered the webbing, rather like the spokes of a wheel. Work for two minutes.

Oesophagus: Using the 'caterpillar' technique, place your working thumb halfway down your hand and walk up between the crease between your index and middle fingers. Repeat this move three times.

Rib pain

Many women experience rib pain during pregnancy, particularly later on.

Why does it happen?

During pregnancy, the ribs can be overstretched by the expanding uterus, which can cause pain if there is any restriction in the spine where the ribs articulate. Rib pain (and heartburn – see above) can also be a result of a restriction in the diaphragm.

What can you do?

Osteopathic treatment can be very helpful in relieving symptoms. Also, bear in mind the following:

- ✿ Be aware of how you are breathing – breathing deep and slow, using the diaphragm, will help to change the baby's position, lessening rib pain and encouraging good blood supply.
- ✿ Sleep on your side with good pillow support.

- ❀ Swimming (front or back crawl) will help to mobilize your thorax and ribs.
- ❀ A simple exercise: standing up, holding a broom above your head, with your arms straight, stretch to the right (to 11 o'clock) and to the left (2 o'clock). Breathe deeply and allow your lower ribs to stretch.

Constipation

Almost every woman will suffer from a degree of constipation during pregnancy, as pregnancy hormones slow down the digestive process and it adapts to your developing baby's needs.

Why does it happen?

Pregnancy hormones, lack of water and a diet lacking in fibre-rich foods are all possible contributory factors to constipation. It's not always easy to drink enough water when you are already running to the loo every two minutes. Progesterone suppositories and iron supplements can also cause constipation.

What can you do?

- ❀ Try to sip room-temperature or warm water throughout the day.
- ❀ Include plenty of fibre-rich foods in your diet, including whole grains, such as porridge oats and brown rice, green leafy vegetables and fruit, especially prunes.
- ❀ Choose whole foods wherever possible, rather than refined or processed foods, as whole foods contain the roughage you need.
- ❀ Lightly cooked foods are easier to digest than raw foods.
- ❀ Steer clear of laxatives unless under direct medical supervision, as these can result in painful contractions of the bowel and disrupt the uterus.
- ❀ Gentle exercise can help get the bowel moving.

Tips by type

Heat type

Dry stools, dry mouth and thirst. You may be feeling hot with night sweats. If the Heat is affecting the Stomach, you may also have a constant strong hunger and/or acid indigestion.

Tongue: Red body and possibly a yellow coat (especially if affecting the Stomach).

Treatment: Cooling foods (see p. 59) and small amounts of food. Increase cooling fruits and vegetables and eat fruits away from main meals. A banana before anything else in the morning may help; or make a banana and linseed smoothie in the morning (blitz a banana, honey and linseeds in a blender with either milk, rice or soya milk).

Check you are not consuming anything too Heating from the foods list on p. 58. Even though you have a strong thirst, remember not to flood the digestive system with lots of cold water which will only interfere with its function. Drink warm water away from mealtimes.

Stagnant type

Pebble-like stools that look like rabbit droppings or larger, but they don't come out in one piece. Lots of belching and your tummy sticks out (not that you would notice this necessarily with all the growth there). You might feel a little bad tempered and even depressed and you might be sighing a lot. Sighing is a way of releasing Qi in the chest that can become stuck because of the things we are not saying or built-up frustrations.

Tongue: Mauve.

Treatment: Stop rushing around trying to do everything and getting frustrated. You need to slow down and give yourself more time. Ask yourself if you are feeling happy and what you need to make things work for you in your coming role. Maybe you are feeling emotionally frustrated and have not been honest with yourself. Stagnation usually has its roots in emotional issues that are unresolved, so give yourself the space to think about the roots of your frustration.

Hot water and lemon or cider vinegar and a little honey in hot water first thing in the morning and before each meal is a great tonic for you. Exercise will also help, so if you are sitting at a desk all day, make time to walk around. (The Qi in the lower abdomen needs to move to shift emotions, so thirty minutes' gentle walking a day is a good idea.)

Blood-Deficient type

Dry stools, tiredness, dizziness, dots in front of your eyes, pale complexion and lips.

Tongue: Pale with pale or slightly orange-tinged sides.

Treatment: Get some rest for half an hour in the afternoon to help nourish your Blood. Include Blood-nourishing foods like dates, dark red or black beans and beetroot, and sprinkle seeds (especially small black ones of any description) over salads, soups, stews and noodles. Prune juice is ideal for you, as it nourishes the Blood *and* is a perfect way to move a dry stool.

Reflexology for constipation

Some people find reflexology helpful in relieving constipation.

Reflex areas to treat

Stomach: Massaging the entire web area between the thumb and forefinger with a 'caterpillar' technique (see p. 335), helps to return the healing energy to the whole stomach area and encourage a normal functioning. Continue until you've covered the webbing, rather like the spokes of a wheel. Work for two minutes.

Colon: (On left hand.) To relieve constipation symptoms and help stimulate the peristaltic movement of the colon, place your thumb on the wrist, underneath your ring finger (fourth finger) and walk halfway up the hand, using the 'caterpillar' technique (see p. 335). Push in and stimulate here, before turning left to walk across the hand, ending up by the fleshy thumb webbing. Repeat three times.

Is the Mind on Board?

In the third trimester, in Chinese medicine we talk of 'harmonizing the Heart' in preparation for becoming a mother. You may feel full of energy and excitement or anything but in perfect harmony, as mood swings and high emotions are experienced by many women during the last few weeks of pregnancy. Take comfort in your friends and family, and seek out those who are calming and who instil in you a sense of confidence to focus on the job ahead.

Talking to other women

The Red Tent by Anita Diamant is a novel that tells the biblical story of Jacob and his sons through the women's experience. The book has an enormous following, probably because it portrays a time in history when women lived and supported one another in a way we can only imagine now.

In the red tent (menstrual hut), each month the women celebrate their femininity and their ability to create and sustain life through their menstrual bleeding. All the women tended to have their period at the same time. They tell stories to each other of fertility, labour and birth and they share in each other's joy and suffering. During the time of their bleed, they are exempt from their duties of caring for the men.

Now no one is suggesting we do this today, but I think it is very valuable for women to spend time together when they can discuss many of the issues that women face. In my early days as a practitioner, I had a patient named Sonia, all of whose labours I attended (all at home, except for one). During her pregnancies, I would go to her house and give her treatment in a room which we called the red tent. We talked about being daughters, becoming mothers and being wives, and the joy and heartache that went with the territory. These times were important to both of us, and I know that much of what we discussed during then sustained us in times of need.

We all experience joy and suffering in life, and spending time supporting one another can bring great comfort. Knowing you are understood is often half the battle.

So I would encourage you to cultivate friendships with other women – start a book club, swap skills, take exercise together and bring woman-to-woman wisdom back into our culture. After all, I think that many of the things women talk about with men are really the domain of women and are issues that most men find difficult to empathize with.

When Sonia's longed-for daughter (after three boys) was due to be born, I had started chemotherapy. By some miracle, however, I was able to attend the birth (her only hospital birth). I was so glad to be there to see the birth of her daughter, and to help her with her fear of having a baby in hospital. And for me, the experience of birth while I faced my own mortality filled me with joy and hope and was incredibly healing.

SONIA'S BIRTH STORY

Life often plays tricks on you. Caterina was three days early; I had prepared for a lovely home birth but my waters had meconium in them, and so it wasn't to be. My husband was in a meeting and I could not get hold of him, so I called my homeopath to come and be with me (so much for being brave), and I called Emma in a panic to 'get me into labour' before I was whisked off to hospital. Emma said she couldn't promise anything, but did her magical acupuncture with which I'd always resonated really well – except I didn't feel anything. I just wasn't going into labour, and I was about to be dragged into hospital. I was packed into the car and raced off to the hospital, wailing and weeping that I could not give birth without my husband being there. He was nowhere to be found, oblivious to the drama that was unfolding.

By the time we reached the hospital, girl power had taken over! My two beautiful birthing partners had got me laughing so hard that I suddenly saw the funny side of things. They put me in a dodgy wheelchair and we bumped our way in fits and starts down the hospital corridors – all I could see were Emma's sparkly shoes dancing beside me. She had just had her first chemotherapy and I was worried about her, but she was determined not to attract attention and she looked like a fairy princess!

I got to the birthing suite, took off my dress, chatted, squatted on the bed, made birthing sounds that I did not recognize as coming from me. At the final moments, I could hear the girls giving me instructions, holding me and giving me their energy to be able to push, and within twenty minutes of arriving at the hospital Caterina was born with the cord wrapped round her neck, but otherwise fine.

The birth was so short I couldn't believe it. What I did not realize was that I had relaxed with my girlfriends and allowed the natural process to take place. I had allowed my true self to give birth, without worrying that I would scare my partner off sex for life, or that he would faint at the sight of the blood. I totally let go for the first time in my life and grabbed the nurturing female energy that literally surrounded me to give me the strength to push the baby out. It was magical, and although I had a pang of guilt, I now know why for centuries the birthing room was a female-dominated area. The energy is just so different.

My husband rushed in as I was getting cleaned up. He was proud to be a father and bonded instantly with our little girl. I do think that I saw a twinkle of relief, mixed with guilt that he preferred to have come in at the end. If I had to repeat the birthing experience, I would say from the outset that I prefer men stay outside the birthing room, and I am sure that secretly they might agree . . .

chapter twelve
PREPARING FOR LABOUR

The end of pregnancy is not a bundle of laughs in terms of comfort. But nature is clever and I remember thinking, 'Just get this baby out of me; bring on labour.' You will be slowing down and if you aren't, I really encourage you to do so. There is so much pressure on women to work right up until they drop, and this means they often enter into labour and motherhood exhausted. If at all possible, try and slow right down from thirty-six weeks. You really will need to prepare mentally for the huge and wondrous event that is ahead of you.

Whenever I am faced with an enormous task, one that involves both physical endurance and mental strength, I apply the same rule: I live in the moment and do only what I can do in the here and now. Never does this rule apply more than in labour.

It is important to try and remain grounded in the here and now of labour, by which I mean dealing only with what is directly in front of you. So in the context of labour, treat every contraction as an isolated incident, rather than in relation to what came before or what will be coming next. Break it down and think, 'I am dealing with this fine' and, 'I can deal with this contraction because it is getting me nearer to my goal.' If your mind and body are calm and strong with it, the midwife will hopefully report back to you that the cervix is opening or becoming more favourable. If, on the other hand, you panic that the most recent contraction was so much more painful then the last one, and you are concerned about the one that's coming next, you will be projecting your energy all over the place, rather than where it is needed: deep inside the pelvis and the cervix. When you come to labour, imagine that with every individual breath, you are opening up gently, like the petals of a flower, and that your body is able to handle each contraction in a strong, yet gentle, way.

*

In the following chapters, you will find ways in which you can help yourself prepare for the amazing job of labour. In *The Red Tent* (see p. 242), it is said that labour is where you learn the courage to be a parent. It will be hard work (it's not called labour for nothing); in fact, it will probably be the hardest thing your body and your mind have had to endure (except, perhaps, for your own birth). But try to be positive.

I also want you to be organized for motherhood and the month following childbirth. To this end, I have included a store cupboard to prepare for the postnatal period (see p. 252). This includes foods that will help in your recovery and also with your breast milk production. Many women cannot see past the labour, which isn't surprising since it is such a momentous event. However, to be prepared is to be calm and able to focus on the important job of looking after your baby. I don't want you to leave the house for at least two weeks, if possible, after the baby is born. (I do understand though that not everyone is in a position to do this, especially if they have other children or are on their own with the new baby.) I also want to discourage you from going to the supermarket where cold air pumped out from the fridges and freezers is the last thing you need having just given birth.

WAYS TO HELP ACHIEVE A NATURAL DELIVERY

- Good posture towards the end of pregnancy is vital to help the position of your baby.
- Avoid sofas and opt for sitting on a ball. Keep your knees lower than your hips.
- Move around freely; walking will help to relax the psoas muscle – a major muscle, responsible for stabilizing the base of the spine.
- Get plenty of rest and build up your energy reserves.
- Make sure the mind is on board – you'll need a heavy dose of mental strength to get through labour.
- Pre-birth acupuncture is excellent for all of the above. In my clinic, we give regular acupuncture as preparation for labour and also teach partners how to do acupressure during labour (see p. 268).

Birth Plan

It's not essential to have a written birth plan, but writing down what you ideally want to happen during your labour and talking it through with the midwife, can be helpful not only for you, but for others, so they know your wishes. It's more a 'birth preferences plan' than something written in stone, as anything can happen and you may need to be open to changes, but it's a great place to start.

By talking through your birth plan you will get to know what's possible or not wherever you are having your baby – for example, whether you can play your own music or when friends and family can visit. Your midwife should incorporate your birth plan into your antenatal notes and it's a good idea to keep a copy tucked in your handbag or hospital bag too.

You can put whatever you like in your birth plan, but here are just a few points that I'd recommend you include:

- ❀ Your preferred delivery position
- ❀ Preferred pain relief options (p. 268)
- ❀ Who will be present at the birth
- ❀ Who you would like to cut the umbilical cord
- ❀ Whether you want your baby placed on your chest immediately after birth; most hospitals will do this now as a matter of course, but it's still useful to check
- ❀ Whether you are keen to have a natural third stage (delivery of the placenta) or would accept drugs to speed up the normal delivery
- ❀ Postnatal-care plan for all the possible outcomes

Pre-birth Acupuncture

Pre-birth acupuncture is a series of acupuncture treatments given in the last few weeks of pregnancy to help prepare the mother for labour. The emphasis of treatment at this stage is to increase Qi and Blood in the woman to help her energy through labour (and in the all-important first few weeks after the birth). Secondly, the treatment is aimed at preparing the cervix and pelvis for labour.

In Germany, many women use acupuncture as a routine part of labour preparation. The research available is promising, showing that the time spent in labour is reduced by just under two hours, and that in the women receiving acupuncture prior to labour there was less intervention.[26]

Acupuncture is inexpensive to give, is safe, normally painless and has proven benefits. I would love to see a day when all women could access it on the NHS. In practice, I really value this time spent with women, it is such a special time and also one when I can talk about the importance of the postnatal period. Some of the conversations I have had with women just before they became mothers are among the most memorable I have been fortunate enough to have. Thoughts of hopes and dreams, fears and doubts, tears for what is being lost, yet what is being gained: laughing through tears, my favourite emotion.

Back Support

Sitting tall in an upright chair that offers good support, particularly towards your due date, will help the baby to maintain the best position for birth; or if you want to, lie down, but always give your baby space. It is believed that the uterus rotates anti-clockwise enabling delivery – a corkscrew effect. The baby will remain long, with the back of its head (occiput) left and the spine in front, in 'pole' position for birth. So if you slump back, your baby can go back-to-back which makes the labour more difficult for both of you.

Take a scarf or something similar with you when you go out, to ensure you can always provide a cushion for your lower back; or, better still, sitting on a foam wedge or on a chair that tilts forward, actively encourages your baby to lie correctly.

Now is the time to walk tall and be proud of your gorgeous bump. Keeping long, maintaining optimum length between your pelvis and ribcage means your baby is able to get into pole position for delivery.

A PRE-LABOUR TIP

Before your due date, put a clean fresh towel under you while you sleep. Take this with you to the hospital to deliver. Then, if you have a Caesarean section, your baby can be put in this towel smelling of you immediately after delivery, providing a much better introduction to you and our world, than a rough hospital towel.

Yoga for Birth

The very best help that yoga can offer you in labour is the capacity to remain completely in the present moment, without the tensions that arise from expectation or fear. This is truly the state of yoga or 'union', and in this state you can act from powerful intuitive understanding of what is right for you and your baby.

There are two essential yoga practices which can help you to remain in this state of openness and acceptance through labour, and it is best to practise them as much as possible throughout your pregnancy, so that you can trust they really work for you.

Sankalpa

The first practice is to establish for yourself a 'sankalpa' or an affirmation that states your heart's deepest desire for this baby and birth. For example: 'I have everything I need to birth my baby well', or, 'My body is totally ready to birth my baby.' The statement should be a closely held secret, to give you courage and strength, and to focus your energies during the birth, keeping you present as the labour unfolds. Take time to discover what the best sankalpa is for you and your baby, then let your own inner voice of wisdom and strength repeat it silently to you on the exhaling breath. It is helpful to use the sankalpa in relaxation practices throughout pregnancy, when you wake up in the morning, as you drift off to sleep and then to hear it repeated on your breath as you labour.

Golden thread breath

Above all other practices, this simple exhalation is the antidote to pain, anxiety and fear during labour. It often arises instinctively in women who are coping well with their labour, so it makes good sense to practise it during pregnancy, so that your body is familiar with the relaxing effects; then it will spontaneously arise when you need it most, without having to be reminded.

You can do this practice in any position, standing, sitting, lying or walking. All you need to do is to breathe in through the nose and out through your mouth. Start softly, with sighs and yawns to release your lips and jaw, then begin with the mouth open quite widely, making a loud sighing sound. As you settle into the rhythm of the breath, let the exhalation lengthen to a comfortable pace, and allow the mouth to be soft and easy, perhaps almost closed, with only a tiny gap between the top and bottom lips. Imagine that there is a golden thread of breath leaving through the lips, and focus the mental attention out on the end of the breath as it floats away. The farther away the breath floats, the more completely the body can relax. The main point of this breath is for it to be effortless, and to create a sense of quiet and easy release, so experiment and play with inhaling through the nose and exhaling through the mouth until you find a balance that suits you. When you are comfortable with the breath, it will feel totally effortless, and deeply calming.

Peaks and valleys/wave crests and troughs

Many women find it really helpful to visualize their labour as a journey – perhaps over the ocean or through the mountains.

The breath leads you through the challenges of the journey, with a steady, sure guidance. The contractions are like giant waves or high mountains that you need to traverse on your journey to motherhood. You can trust that the breath will always lead you over the next peak or across the next wave, because you can always hold your focus on 'just one more breath'.

During the first stage of labour, it can be very useful to alternate the golden thread breath (described above) with *ujayii* breath (described on p. 196) to carry you through the journey. For example, as you exhale, feel the golden thread exhalation like it's a steady rope leading you up the paths to the tops of the mountains or over the crests of the waves, and then down the other side. When you come to rest in the valleys, or the troughs between the waves (which represent the spaces between the contractions), then revert to *ujayii* breath. Use *ujayii* as a resting breath, and take the time to gather your resources, nourishing yourself with the breath in between the great surges of uterine energy in the contractions. Practise this alternating of breaths for a whole minute, to mimic the length of the average contraction: up and down the mountains or waves with golden thread exhalation, and then peacefully down in the valleys, resting with *ujayii* breath.

Moving with ease, breathing freely

Revisit the cat poses (see p. 204) in preparation for birth, and explore how comfortable you feel opening out the pelvis by stepping one foot off your mat to the side, knee bent. Place your hands on the floor and circle freely in both directions. Breathe easily, practising golden thread breath as you move.

Then bring your foot back to the starting place, step the other side and repeat again. This half-squat position is a sustainable and realistic alternative to a full squat, and has the advantage of being a position in which you can move freely with an open pelvis. It is an ideal birthing position for many women. Practise moving freely from this position back to the cat pose, and then experiment with resting forwards on a chair seat and rocking to and fro to find what feels most comfortable for you. Breathe freely throughout your movements.

Birthing breath

When labour moves into the second stage, and your baby is ready to be born, there is a palpable shift in energy as your whole being readies itself to birth your baby. At this point, many women find they vocalize the most deep and powerful 'lowing' sounds, as if their breath were calling their babies into the world. From a yoga perspective, it makes sense to harness this instinctive use of breath, so that it can provide you with as much assistance as possible. Recall the pelvic-floor practices (see p. 206) and sense how the powerful exhalation can be directed to 'breathe the baby down'. It is as if now you direct the whole of your energies and breathe into the birth canal, breathing the baby down through the vagina. Let the jaw and mouth be soft and open, and the exhalation long and free, perhaps carrying out deep sounds. It is crucial to allow for the pelvic floor to release and relax completely, and to hold no tension that might obstruct the passage of the baby. Free movement, perhaps in the cat-pose variations (see p. 204) or the half-squat options (described in the previous section) can ensure that the pelvis is well open and the baby well positioned, so that a powerful breath can encourage their long-awaited arrival. Remember that with every breath you come one step closer to meeting your baby.

For more information on Uma Dinsmore-Tuli's books and website, and yoga in pregnancy, please see Resources, p. 339, and Further Reading, p. 347.

Preparing Your Postnatal Store Cupboard

The emphasis here is on building Qi and Blood. Stock up on:

❀ Rice
❀ Oats (cooked in porridge rather than uncooked in muesli)

❀ Corn
❀ Kidney beans
❀ Adzuki beans
❀ Sweet potatoes
❀ Yams
❀ Squash
❀ Mushrooms
❀ Leafy green vegetables
❀ Spinach
❀ Beetroot
❀ Eggs
❀ Red meat
❀ Sesame seeds (black, if you can find them)
❀ *Herbs*
  • Ginger
  • Cinnamon
  • Fenugreek
  • Nutmeg
  • Rosemary
  • Basil
  • Cloves
  • Fennel seeds (for cooking and tea)
  • Dill
  • Thyme
❀ Jasmine tea
❀ *Snacks*
  • Apricots
  • Dates
  • Sesame-seed bars
  • Liquorice
  • Ginger biscuits
  • Soups
  • Chocolate beetroot cake (see recipe, p. 310)

Preparation tips

❀ Order your organic delivery box (see Resources, p. 342) in advance.

❀ Prepare your chicken stock (see recipe below) and freeze in batches for making soup.

Chicken stock

You can make chicken stock with a single uncooked chicken carcass (see p. 303) or use a roast chicken carcass, as described here.

Pull any of the spare meat and set aside. Next, push down on the carcass until you hear the bones crack, then pull it apart and add to a large stockpot. Use the entire carcass, including any juices left in the roasting pan.

Add to the stockpot:
2 large carrots, chopped
2 cloves
2 celery stalks
2 bay leaves
2 onions, halved with skins left on
sprig of thyme
10 peppercorns

1. Cover the ingredients with fresh water and bring almost to the boil. Reduce the heat and keep at a low simmer for 1½–2 hours. Check intermittently and skim off any froth that rises to the surface.
2. Cool and strain the stock through a fine sieve. Freeze for later use.

ALL THE TEA IN CHINA

A patient of mine, Alice, told me about her experience with raspberry-leaf tea.

Alice was thirty-nine weeks pregnant. Ten members of her family had met up for Sunday lunch. In the morning, they had gone on a three-mile walk and then, being the middle of winter, they had settled down to a boozy, long lunch.

Alice found she could not sit down at the table for long and kept getting up throughout the meal to make herself pots of fresh raspberry-leaf tea. It was, she said, like a little meditation and gave her a breathing space away from the jolly chattering around the table. Back and forth she went to the kitchen; she estimated that over the course of the three-hour lunch, she must have made four trips to the kitchen to refill her teapot.

That night, Alice awoke with labour pains. Things had well and truly started and she knew that this was it. Samuel was born – a healthy 3.6kg baby – before breakfast the next morning. Alice puts her efficient labour down to the three-mile walk, her little pilgrimages to the kitchen and the powers of raspberry-leaf tea!

I think it is always better to drink the loose-leaf variety and to drink several cups, not just one tea bag per day. Perhaps not quite as much as Alice, but in her case, I think the tea served as an escape as much as anything else.

And for those of you who were looking forward to not drinking it once labour is through – it is a brilliant postnatal tonic too!

Fear and Labour

There is a never-ending list of things that you could be afraid of during pregnancy and in labour: 'Will I cope?' 'Will it be painful?' 'Will I be all right?' 'Will the baby be all right?' The list goes on and on. But fear is there for a reason. It is part of our survival instinct; it is our will to survive and reproduce. It's that rush of adrenalin or Kidney energy that gives us the power we need to run from tigers, reproduce, keep going when we want to stop and, *yes* – survive labour. It is one of our deepest instincts, and without it, we probably would not have evolved to where we are today.

The problem is that when fear takes over, it can seriously weaken us emotionally and physically. Just as we are getting tired and there are a few chinks in our armour, out come the scaremongers – people in the street, healthcare professionals, friends and work colleagues – merchants of doom (albeit well-intentioned) are everywhere: 'Oh that baby looks big.' 'How many weeks did you say you were?'

'Well, of course, I laboured for three days before they discovered the baby was breech.' 'I practically had mine in the corridor.'

You'll need to protect yourself from people's negativity. It's really important. Focus on keeping your strength and not giving in to fear. If you choose to engage in these images and focus on the negative, you are more likely to invite that outcome – it is the law of attraction. And in case you think I have gone all crystals and feathers on you, I do have a bit of science to back this up.

Adrenalin, which we produce when we are afraid, neutralizes oxytocin, a hormone which plays a vital role during labour (see p. 265). So fear gets in the way of having good, strong contractions. Similarly, in Chinese medicine the Kidneys are needed to supply the emotional and physical stamina required for labour. Good, strong Kidney Qi means that you have appropriate fear – enough to get you through labour and some left over for afterwards. Weak Kidney Qi means ineffectual contractions, prolonged labour, fear of pain and, ultimately, a long labour and shattered mum afterwards.

I encourage you to seek out positive stories of birth. My mother always taught me that her labours were the biggest achievements of her life. The pain was unspoken and only the pride remained.

Facing your fears

✿ Have a good look in the mirror and identify what it is you fear.
✿ Ask yourself what you need to overcome your fears.
✿ Choose a positive statement about how you wish your labour to be, or how you wish to manage the task ahead of you.
✿ Choose what physical and mental attribute you need to be with you as you go into labour. Be creative. You may decide you need the courage of a lion or you may feel humour is more important. I had a friend who amused us between contractions and kept us all in stitches. She had a very straightforward home birth. You may decide that you need a secret painkilling breath that no one in the world but you has discovered yet. Whatever it is, work on it before labour and draw on these thoughts and images whenever you need them.

❀ Rest. Don't exhaust yourself running around the shops in the last days of pregnancy or working out in the gym. Yes, it's good to be fit, but not exhausted.

Of course, with the best will in the world, things don't always turn out the way we want or imagine that they will and that can be disappointing. As long as you can feel you did your best though, you will easily resolve any feelings of disappointment.

One last word on fear: I believe that the things we fear the most are the places in our lives where we stand the most to learn about ourselves and our abilities. When you view fear in this way, it ceases to be a threat, and can be a teacher instead.

CASE STUDY

MEGAN'S HOME BIRTH USING THE BIRTHING POOL

When I [Anna] arrived it was clear that Megan's labour had started. The contractions were now 2:10. Megan was on her bed on all fours where she felt most comfortable. By 1 a.m., the contractions had increased to 3:10, and to touch they felt strong. Megan felt all of the pain from the contractions in her back and felt the most comfortable on her hands and knees and leaning against the pillows and headboard at the top of her bed. Megan wasn't losing any more fluid and the baby's heartbeat was good.

Megan coped really well with the rapidly increasing pain, using breathing techniques and changing her position and walking around. Her partner decided to fill the pool and Megan was very happy to immerse herself in the warm water. 'My body did not feel heavy, I had more freedom to move and a great feeing of weightlessness. I felt I could properly relax between contractions and let myself go. It was my space. People couldn't get too close to me and this gave me freedom, as I was in control to be in the position I wanted to be in without having to rely on people for support.'

Megan's contractions continued to become stronger. Unusually, she felt them all in her lower back. She got some relief from her partner or me massaging her lower back. Megan stretched out on her back in the pool between contractions and sucked ice cubes to keep herself cool and hydrated.

As the contractions became stronger, Megan spent more time on her knees, leaning over the edge of the pool. This way she could rest and be upright at the same time. She could flop forward between contractions, and relax her head on the side.

At about 4.30 p.m., Megan felt she'd hit a brick wall and wasn't making any more progress. The back pain was even more intense, and no matter how hard we massaged to counterbalance the pain of the contractions in her back, Megan felt exhausted. We had a discussion, and decided I would do a vaginal examination and break her waters. Megan got out of the pool for this procedure.

The baby's position was good and there had been descent of the head. The baby's heartbeat was strong. Megan was 9.5cm and I ruptured her waters easily. Megan had a contraction out of the pool and it was much more intense and painful for her without the analgesic and relaxing properties of the warm water, so she quickly got back in.

The second midwife arrived at this time with some entonox, which Megan tried but didn't like as she felt it took her control away. She felt focused through her breathing and the help of the water. The pain had changed, and Megan felt a 'mental switch' between the first and second stage of labour. She felt 'she could do it' and that the hardest bit was over.

As Megan entered the second stage of labour, she began to feel an involuntary urge to push. She needed no encouragement from me; she felt directed by her body's response to the natural progression of labour. 'I felt physically very strong with a renewed energy. This motivated me to push as hard as I could.'

A short time later, the baby began to crown. One push and her head came out, and then a short break until the next contraction, when Megan pushed her baby out. She was in the water and I passed her through Megan's legs. Megan picked her up, elated and exhausted. She sat back and leant against the edge of the pool to admire her gorgeous baby.

(Megan's story from Anna)

Roots – visualization for late pregnancy and early labour

You know how it is when a plant has grown too big for its pot and you need to re-pot it, so it can continue to thrive and grow? When the roots leave the soil, and the tension falls away from them, as they are released from the light grasp of the earth, giving them an easy, comfortable pathway and a safe journey to their new environment? How you just know when that precious jewel you have watched over and nurtured is ready to emerge – when the time is right? As with the seasons, sometimes there is a longer winter and a shorter spring and you wonder if winter will ever end. But you know it must, at just the right time.

As you feel the excitement stirring within you, knowing that when the time is right spring will begin, you can trust your unconscious mind with the knowledge that many generations of mothers before you have experienced this time easily and naturally too, to allow you to be here now. You can trust your unconscious mind to choose exactly the right time for you to change seasons and move towards spring, with energy and brightness. You know that your body is made to give birth when the time is right, and you can trust that.

And just for a moment, I'd like you to imagine your mother, grandmothers and the long line of women whose skills at childbirth have brought you to today, and to the baby growing inside you. Know that without them, and their expertise and experience, you would not be here. Notice how easily and calmly they pass their combined knowledge on to you, so that you too can benefit from it. Tap into that massive pool of experience and take whatever lessons you need from it, to further enhance your baby's birth in a way that is both safe and natural. Take a moment to thank your ancestors for creating you, and for contributing to the life within you, and know that by giving birth to your own baby, only when the time is right and safe to do so, you too will belong to this amazing fountain of knowledge, adding your own to that deep pool.

part four
BIRTH

Labour is a part of nature, and yet the experience can vary a great deal from one woman to the next. You'd think the signs of labour would be hard to miss, and that's true for most women, although some may feel little more than a few twinges in the early stages. This is why I put so much emphasis on preparing your body and your mind for labour and, of course, what comes after. You can't control 100 per cent of what happens, just as in life, but you can be prepared, which will help you stay positive and relaxed, as far as possible.

> *Women must rely on what they feel, rather than what they read or what they were told. To encourage a woman to eat noodles or to add honey to her tea is no more appropriate than it is to impose restrictions. The only recommendation we can make is to avoid making recommendations.*
> Michel Odent, The Caesarean

Labour is a time when a woman must be guided by her intuition and not rely on books or lengthy advice from others. It is far better for a woman to be left to find her own way with gentle guidance, than to be given direct instructions or to be asked too many questions. Labour will show her what to do.

chapter thirteen
EARLY LABOUR

The person who removes a mountain begins by carrying away small stones.
Chinese proverb

There are three stages of labour. The start of labour is defined as when you are having regular contractions and your cervix is 3cm or more dilated – almost a third of the way. The build-up to even this first stage is gradual for most women and, to confuse matters, you might experience Braxton Hicks contractions in the days or weeks ahead of labour.

The second stage of labour begins when your cervix is fully – i.e. 10cm – dilated. This is the stage where you push, and on average, it lasts around two hours. The second stage finale is the birth, and the third stage happens after your baby is born, during which the placenta and membranes are delivered, either naturally or managed with drugs.

Braxton Hicks Contractions

Your body does its own preparation work for labour and delivery, and Braxton Hicks contractions are a part of this process. When you have a Braxton Hicks contraction, your uterus contracts and while you might feel a bit of discomfort, you shouldn't feel pain. They will usually be occasional, rather than regular, but if you do feel any pain, let your midwife know, as you might be going into labour.

Pre-labour

Some women experience a longer period of pre-labour than others, for whom it goes by unnoticed. There may be contractions, perhaps mild and regular, or ones that come in short waves and then stop for a while.

False Labour

False labour is often very difficult to tell apart from the real thing, and occurs more in second and subsequent pregnancies. It can be pretty frustrating, as the contractions might be strong and painful and may come for several hours before abruptly stopping. The contractions tend to be shorter and cause pain in the lower abdomen, rather than the uterus, but that's not so easy to spot when you're in the middle of them.

SIGNS OF LABOUR

- **A 'show'** This is a mucous, bloody discharge that comes away as your cervix stretches and softens in preparation for labour and delivery. It can happen several days before labour, so isn't considered a definitive sign, but shows that things are happening.
- **Spontaneous breaking of waters** For many women, their waters don't break until delivery is close, but for others they may break up to forty-eight hours before labour. Your midwife may be concerned once you reach twenty-four hours after your waters breaking and haven't yet gone into labour as there can be a risk of infection.
- **An ache or pressure in the lower back or up inside the vagina** Depending on the position of your baby, you may feel a dull ache or pressure, which can be an early sign that labour may come soon. It's not time to alert the midwife yet, but good to be aware that contractions may soon follow.
- **Regular painful contractions** If you are at all worried, however early on in labour, call your midwife or the hospital. If you feel fairly relaxed, call when the contractions are about ten minutes apart, regular and painful.

You'll be asked how the contractions feel, how far apart they are and how long they are lasting, as well as whether your waters have broken and what colour they are, how you are feeling generally and if the baby has been moving normally.

Note: If you are experiencing some contractions but still getting hungry and eating, you might not quite be in labour yet, but just gearing up, as sometimes a woman needs food for active labour to establish itself. Labour is often 'timed' from too early on in the process, which then leads to concerns later on that the labour has been going too long for too little progress.

Early Labour

During early labour, you should be able to sleep or be fairly active in between contractions, depending on whether it is night or daytime. Rest as you need, and eat and drink as you want to, as your body prepares for the next stages of labour. If you have planned a hospital birth, stay at home for as long as is practical and possible, so that you can remain in a relaxed environment; research has shown that the more relaxed women are, the better the outcomes on average.

Contractions

Contractions are a sensation caused by muscles at the top of your uterus which contract and radiate downwards towards the cervix, pressing down on your baby and pulling up your cervix, so that it opens. They are usually described in wave-like terms, building up gradually to a peak, then fading to nothing again. As labour progresses, the contractions become stronger, but gradually so, and your body is able to adjust and cope, especially if you are feeling mentally prepared.

It will depend on your own circumstances, and what you have discussed with your midwife or doctor, but usually it's recommended you go to the hospital (unless you are having a home birth, of course) when your contractions are lasting around forty-five seconds and are about three to five minutes apart.

Coping with early labour pain at home

There is a suggestion that animals seem less distressed by labour because they lack the capacity to imagine what might happen or how long the labour might take, they literally cope with one contraction at a time. There's much to be said for developing strategies that help to mirror this, focusing on the moment and relaxing in between the contractions either by pottering around, resting, making cups of tea or having a bath.

Acupressure for early labour

If the membranes have ruptured: acupressure points Sp 6, Li 4, Bl 32 (see p. 269).

OXYTOCIN

Oxytocin is affectionately termed the 'love hormone', as it is released when we connect lovingly with others, even through simple touch. Oxytocin can make us feel more generous, trusting and bring us closer to others. It's wonderful for our emotional health.

Oxytocin is made in the foetus and placenta, and released to help trigger labour contractions. It also stimulates the release of milk for breast-feeding; levels rise when you touch or even look at your newborn baby. Studies have found that massage can stimulate the release of oxytocin, so your partner giving you a massage during the early stages of labour can be extremely beneficial.

TENS

TENS stands for transcutaneous electrical nerve stimulation and is, basically, a little hand-held device attached to four pads by wires, which gives out small pulses of electrical energy. It's not entirely clear why these little pulses can help with pain, but for many women, it's a very helpful non-invasive, drug-free form of pain relief during labour.

The key is to start using the machine as soon as your labour begins, as it takes about an hour for your body to respond and release the endorphins which act as pain relievers. You, or ideally your partner, place the pads according to the instructions on your back, two under the bra line and two just above your bottom, either side of the spine.

Initially, you start on a low setting, then boost during contractions, turning off again after the contraction passes. You can't use the machine if you are having a water birth, but can use it before and after, and many women find TENS helpful in alleviating afterbirth and post-Caesarean pains. Very few hospitals automatically provide TENS machines and they are more effective if you start to use the machine in early labour, so if you're keen to try this method, you can rent or buy a machine for home use, then take it with you into the hospital.

Here are some of the most frequently asked questions about using TENS machines:

Q. It's an electrical current. Is it really harmless?
A. Yes. Women have been using TENS in childbirth for decades, and there have been no recorded side effects on either mother or baby.

Q. I reckon it's just a placebo. What does it actually do?
A. TENS encourages the body to release endorphins, which are natural pain-relieving chemicals (the body's equivalent of morphine). It also targets the pain gate, which stops pain signals from reaching the brain.

Q. I'm booked in for an epidural/Caesarean/water birth. There's no point, is there?
A. Epidurals, Caesarean sections and getting into the water don't take place until relatively late in the labouring process. TENS will offer pain relief until this point, where there is little else on offer (in particular at home) for the early stages.

> *Only when you can be extremely pliable and soft*
> *can you be extremely hard and strong.*
> Zen proverb

chapter fourteen
ADVANCED LABOUR AND BIRTH

At between 8 and 10cm dilation, women go into 'transition'. At this stage, the body makes the transition from drawing up the cervix to beginning to receive messages to bear down, in order to give birth. Some women feel quite confused at this point, many feel angry or upset or want to leave, or feel, as Michel Odent, the legendary obstetrician, puts it, like 'going to another planet'. Make sure your partner knows this might happen, as it's often the point where women swear, scream and push people away, or demand pain-relief drugs that they were keen to avoid. One woman I laboured with said she had had enough and wanted to go home; half an hour later the baby was born.

Ideally, at this point, your midwife will say as little as possible, and not ask you any specific questions like the last time you went to the loo, as your neocortex has very deliberately reduced its activity to help you through the birth.

Dim lights are a very good idea in labour, as bright lights, like questions, will stimulate your neocortex, which you don't need right now. You may also appreciate as much privacy at this time as possible, as a sense of 'being observed' may be too stimulating at a time when you need to feel as secure and relaxed as possible.

The contractions change in the second stage from being waves that you try to breathe through as they peak and disappear, to being sensations that you start to push with.

Pain Relief

Pain relief during labour can come in many forms, so it is very helpful to know your options ahead of time so that you can make your own individual and informed choices. I have included acupressure techniques for early labour and explain the various medical pain-relief options. The key here is to maintain open dialogue and communication with your midwife and caregivers, so that you receive the best care (which includes pain relief) for you and your baby.

Acupressure

In my early days as an acupuncturist, I would attend labours, giving acupuncture as pain relief. However, as I had my own children, and my practice got busier, it became more difficult to attend labours, and I began to encourage the partners to come along to the last few pre-birth acupuncture treatments, so that I could teach them some basic acupressure points. This became very popular and I soon started holding small classes to teach small groups of couples.

Having received feedback from many couples, I now believe that the combination of pre-birth acupuncture and acupressure during labour is actually better than using acupuncture in labour. It allows the woman far more movement and is far less invasive; it also cuts down the amount of people in the birthing room. And, most importantly, it allows the partner to be involved. But be aware that there are no prizes for not accepting stronger pain relief if that is what is required.

Tips for using acupressure in labour – for partners
- ❀ Start early on in labour, before the pains have intensified.
- ❀ Some points will feel good to receive and some not so good, so ask for feedback.
- ❀ The points should not actually feel unpleasant or overly painful; if they do, try applying less pressure, then gradually increasing as your partner is able to tolerate more.
- ❀ Don't be unrealistic; acupressure can help promote a more efficient labour and it is a useful tool to move things along, but don't

expect that your partner will suddenly be pain-free. This is labour and the pain is there for a reason.

Acupressure for labour

Bl 67 (Bladder 67)

Using ear-press seeds on Bl 67 is a useful tool to try and encourage the baby into the right position during labour. Using seeds to stimulate these points (attached with a plaster) may encourage the baby into a more comfortable position for you. See p. 227 for an illustration of where point Bl 67 is located.

Sp 6 (Spleen 6)

- ❀ Apply firm pressure with thumbs or index finger.
- ❀ Use on one leg at a time for one minute.

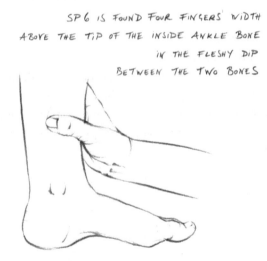

SP 6 IS FOUND FOUR FINGERS' WIDTH ABOVE THE TIP OF THE INSIDE ANKLE BONE IN THE FLESHY DIP BETWEEN THE TWO BONES

Bl 60 (Bladder 60)

- ❀ Depression on inside ankle, between the tip of ankle bone and Achilles tendon.
- ❀ Apply pressure with thumbs or by squeezing between thumb and fingers.

❀ Increases the descending function, helping the baby move further down the birth canal.

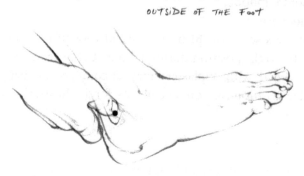

B160 IS FOUND BEHIND THE ANKLE BONE ON THE OUTSIDE OF THE FOOT

THIS POINT IS HELPFUL IF THE BABY IS POSTERIOR AND CAUSING BACK PAIN. COMBINES WELL WITH P6

Li 4 (Large intestine 4)

❀ Main point for pain relief.
❀ Useful for transition and second stage of labour to give the woman the final energy to push the baby out.
❀ Good early on in labour to help establish strong contractions.
❀ An ice cube can be used to apply the pressure, or you can use your thumbs.

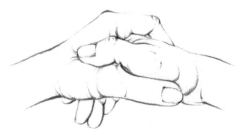

LI4 IS IN THE FLESHY MOUND BETWEEN THUMB AND FIRST FINGER. A REALLY USEFUL POINT IN LABOUR AS IT ENCOURAGES DOWNWARD MOVEMENT

Kid 1 (Kidney 1)

- ❀ Apply pressure with thumb or knuckles angled up towards the big toe.
- ❀ Sometimes used with sea-sickness bands, allowing the woman to walk around while the ball on the bands applies pressure to the point on the foot.
- ❀ Very calming; good for anxiety and to help with panic especially during the transition period.

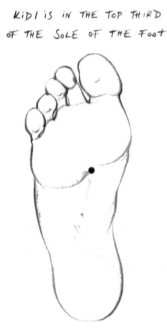

KID1 IS IN THE TOP THIRD
OF THE SOLE OF THE FOOT

USE YOUR KNUCKLE TO STIMULATE
THE POINT, PUSHING UPWARDS
TOWARDS THE TOES

Hand points

There is a row of points on the palm of the hand, in the crease where the fingers meet the hand. These points can be stimulated by the woman wrapping her fingers around a comb or by the partner squeezing the base of each finger, applying small circular movements.

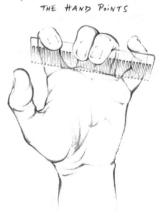

GRIP A COMB to STIMULATE
THE HAND POINTS

PRESSURE ON THESE HAND POINTS
WILL RELEASE ENDORPHINS
To HELP YOU COPE WITH THE PAIN

Bl 32 (Bladder 32)

❀ This point lies between the dimples and the spine above the buttocks, in a small dip on the sacrum (which is actually a small hole in the underlying bone).

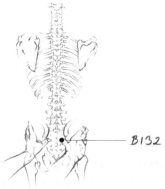

Bl32 IS GOOD FOR BACK PAIN

APPLYING PRESSURE TO THESE POINTS
(ON EITHER SIDE OF THE SPINE)
WILL PROVIDE RELIEF IN LABOUR

Bl32

- ❈ Apply pressure with the knuckles or thumbs.
- ❈ The function can be intensified by the woman leaning back into the partner's knuckles or by the woman rocking.
- ❈ Strengthens the intensity of the contractions and helps alleviate back pain.

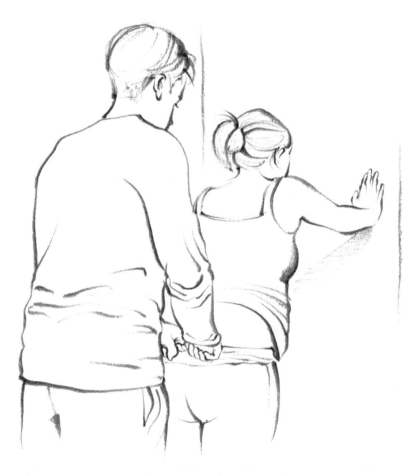

Gb 21 (Gall Bladder 21)

- ❀ Located at the highest point of the shoulder muscle.
- ❀ Pressure needs to be applied from above.
- ❀ Helps descent and to stimulate contractions.

USE GB21 DURING CONTRACTIONS
TO HELP STIMULATE THE UTERUS

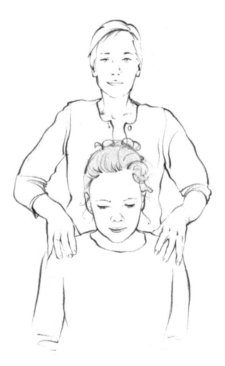

THIS POINT IS GREAT IN FIRST AND
SECOND STAGE LABOUR. USE THUMBS OR EVEN
FOREARMS TO STIMULATE THE POINT

Leading obstetric acupuncturist Debra Betts has produced a fantastic booklet and DVD on acupressure for labour. For more information, see Further Reading, p. 347.

EASING THE PAIN OF LABOUR

I remember one labour I attended when I used acupressure and homeopathy to help the labouring woman. She was getting a great deal of backache: 'My back, my back,' she kept repeating over and over. This had been going on for an hour, and I could see it was tiring her out. I used the point BI 32 on the lower back and a remedy for backache.

Within minutes of me giving the remedy (and about three minutes of acupressure), she started saying, 'My belly, my belly.' I took this as a sign that what I had done had worked; although she was still in some discomfort, the pain had clearly moved, and she was getting a reprieve from the backache. Mentally, I saw a change in her – I think she viewed the change in the pain as a sign of progression and this was encouraging.

Sometimes, it is as much about changing the energy and the nature of the pain, as it is about getting rid of it. The pain is necessary; if the pain stops, then the labour will stop. But where there is movement there is progress.

A DAD'S EXPERIENCE

'Well, my anecdotal experience when talking to other women before we had any babies was that the worst thing you can do is to dispense any advice during labour. Men tend to read a couple of paragraphs in a baby book and then believe that they are qualified to give out advice and instructions, which most women find, at least annoying, and more likely, grounds for physical violence during labour!

My own experience is that I wanted my wife to know I was supporting her all the way through, whatever that meant. So if that was helping with gas and air or squeezing hands or just talking, then that was fine. Be led by your partner. She is unlikely to be slow in telling you what she needs, and you are there to help with whatever that might be. Also, labour can be a much longer experience than you might think, before you get to the classic delivery time which we have all seen in films. It is important during those long hours to help with relaxation and comfort and calm. Radio 4 also helps!'

Medical pain relief and intervention

Ask your midwife or doctor to talk through the pain-relief options with you ahead of time, and make your wishes clear in your birth plan, while remaining aware that you might need to be flexible on the actual day, according to circumstances.

Epidural

This is a nerve-blocking drug that is injected into the epidural space inside the vertebrae. Ideally, an epidural will take away the pain without taking away sensation, although it can cause a feeling of heaviness in the legs in some women, impairing their ability to move around. The timing of epidurals is important; they are not usually used until established labour and not used if labour is too close to the second stage when the woman needs to push. Once the epidural has been set up, the drugs can be given in a constant drip infusion or topped up by the midwife when needed. Many hospitals do offer very low-dose epidurals now, so that the woman's ability to bear down isn't lost, but if the epidural has been topped up quite a lot then this can happen.

Epidurals may result in a slightly longer labour, as the second stage may be more prolonged if the mother has no significant urge to push. This may increase the likelihood of intervention, such as an oxytocin drip, or assisted delivery.

Gas and air

Gas and air, often known as laughing gas, is inhaled through a self-administered hand-held mask during contractions. It has no effect on the baby and no residual effect on you as soon as you stop breathing it. Some women find it helps to take the edge off the peak of the contractions. Not all women find it helpful, but it will always be on hand if you want to try it.

Injections

Pain-relief drugs, such as pethidine or diamorphine, can be injected into the muscle to help you relax, and therefore lessen the pain. These take about twenty minutes to take effect and last between two and four hours. Some women do feel sick after these injections and, if administered close to the time of delivery, they can affect the ability to push. In some cases, the baby's breathing may be affected, but if that is the case, an antidote can be given. Taking these drugs during labour may also delay the establishment of breastfeeding.

Assisted delivery

If the second stage of labour isn't progressing, you may be offered assistance. Your midwife will be carefully monitoring how effective your contractions are and how your baby is doing. They may check for signs of distress and, if they feel it is the best course of action, talk to you about assisting with an episiotomy (a cut to the vagina to allow the baby's head to pass). If necessary, the midwife may ask an obstetrician to review the progress of labour and they may discuss assisting the delivery, using forceps (which are like large tongs and used to cradle the baby's head), Ventouse (a suction method to help the baby move down the birth canal) or, in some cases, an emergency Caesarean section.

Caesarean section

A Caesarean section can be elective (where you are booked in for the operation) or an emergency (due to complications in labour). Caesareans are almost always performed under a regional anaesthetic (epidural or spinal), so that you will be awake and the baby is delivered through a surgical incision in the abdomen and uterine wall.

Reasons for an elective Caesarean section include:

- ❀ a condition such as pre-eclampsia (see p. 221)
- ❀ diabetes
- ❀ the baby not developing properly in the womb (intrauterine growth restriction)
- ❀ the baby being in a difficult position (see Breech, p. 226)
- ❀ twins or multiple births
- ❀ placanta praevia
- ❀ previous Caesarean section.

Reasons for an emergency Caesarean section include:

- ❀ vaginal bleeding or placental abruption (where the placenta partially or completely separates from the lining of the uterus)

- ❀ the baby's heart rate slowing or being erratic
- ❀ failure to progress in labour
- ❀ cord prolapse (where the cord comes through the cervix ahead of the baby).

Having a Caesarean is no easy option. It is major surgery and usually involves a longer hospital stay. Women who have had a Caesarean also need to be particularly careful with their recovery, both physically and emotionally. Ideally, the decision to perform a Caesarean is taken with you swiftly, and as soon as the baby shows signs of distress, the priority being to avoid the greater risks of an emergency operation. But of course, emergency Caesarean sections do happen and are for the vast majority very safe. Recovery is different from a vaginal birth, so make sure your wishes for this are covered in your birth plan and that you get good information for both the first twenty-four hours and the following weeks (see p. 287).

First Few Hours After Delivery

If you give birth in hospital, you should still be with your baby for the first twenty-four hours, be given privacy and be able to rest or eat and drink whenever you need to. The length of your hospital stay is your choice, and you can talk to your healthcare team at any point about this, whether you want to go home or don't feel well or confident enough just yet.

Your blood pressure will be checked, you should pass urine within a few hours and you'll be encouraged to move around a bit in normal circumstances. In the first twenty-four hours you should also have your own postnatal care plan, tailored by your healthcare team and you to suit your own and your baby's needs.

A small number of babies develop jaundice, which causes a yellowish colour to the skin and eyes, and should be checked immediately. Likewise, babies who don't pass the greenish-brown meconium (first poo) within twenty-four hours should also be checked straight away.

THE BEST THING I EVER ATE

With my first child, I went into labour at 38 weeks +4 days at my in-laws' house, in the early hours of Boxing Day morning. It was a misty morning and I woke at about 3 a.m. with labour pains.

I woke my sleeping husband and Anna, my sister-in-law (the midwife), and together we decided to make the journey to Chelsea and Westminster.

Beautiful Lily was born in the water by seven that morning, and Roger proudly phoned his sleeping parents to tell them the news. No one had heard us leave, or even knew that three of the party were missing. So when Roger announced (over the phone) to his sleepy father that he was a grand-father for the first time, he actually thought he was joking and playing a trick from the upstairs bedroom!

Meanwhile, in the hospital, having had a very straightforward delivery, I was sent home to our house in London. The cupboards were bare, and I had that strange feeling that although I was ravenous, I just could not put my finger on what it was that I wanted to eat. That afternoon, my in-laws arrived, and Brenda (my mother-in-law) had made me a huge pot of turkey broth. To this day, it is the most delicious and nourishing thing I have ever eaten. As I ate it, I felt every mouthful make me stronger and more able to cope. I can't imagine what I would have been fed if I had been in hospital, but that soup was like some sort of energy-giving elixir. Now I always try to make a pot of soup for friends after they give birth, or if they are in hospital, I try and take some good food in for them.

part five

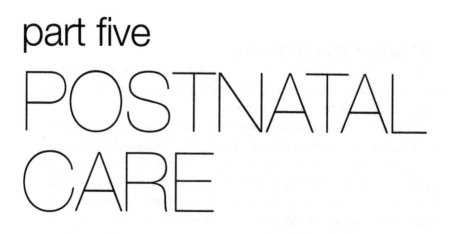

POSTNATAL CARE

This is the most incredible feeling – my favourite part; and while there can be a tendency to almost separate pregnancy from motherhood, they are, of course, intrinsically and intimately linked, on both physical and emotional levels. Pregnancy is really a period of preparation for motherhood, and it is at this crucial, special time, after you have given birth that your health can take a turn for the better or, occasionally, worse. Your physical potential is at its strongest, but you are also at your most vulnerable. Likewise, many women experience bittersweet feelings – of intense love, but also intense fear. This is why my number-one prescription, above all other things, is to take time to rest and recover your energy after giving birth and adjust to your new life. If you, as we say in Chinese medicine, 'do the month' properly (see next chapter), it will pay wonderful dividends later; cut corners, and it may make you more vulnerable to illness later on.

You have now met your longed-for baby and, as you stare into each other's eyes, a new relationship forms that is unique to each parent and child. It may seem daunting, but it is just as it should be, and each mother finds her own way to suit herself and her baby.

chapter fifteen
DOING THE MONTH

There is an expectation in the Western world today that you can rush back into 'normal' life as quickly as you are physically able after giving birth. However, despite the arrival of Western medicine and industrialization in China, millions of women today still follow many of the traditions of 'doing the month'. I encourage all my patients to embrace this wisdom; perhaps it will even become fashionable again, because in my experience the benefits are immeasurable.

As you know from previous chapters, I encourage you to spend time thinking about and preparing for motherhood well ahead of going into labour. For many women, it can come as quite a shock, both physically and emotionally. You will need to give yourself time and space to get used to having a new person in your life who depends on you for food, comfort and love. In Chinese medicine, baby and mother are even treated as one person for the first six months, the connection is that strong.

In 2010, the National Childbirth Trust published a survey into how new mothers feel about the postnatal care given here in the UK. Only 41 per cent of women in the survey felt they received the emotional care they needed in the first twenty-four hours after giving birth. And a third felt they received little or no emotional care in the first month. More than half the women had had assisted deliveries and the gap in postnatal care for operative deliveries was even greater than natural births, and especially for Caesarean births. Many women felt they lacked information on how to feed their baby and general information about their baby's health. All in all, the impact of this lack of perceived care on women's confidence to cope and adjust to motherhood was considered significant, to say the least.[27]

In the following chapters, I provide practical postnatal-care advice, from nutrition to breastfeeding, and hope also to give you confidence and comfort. Enlist your partner and the women around you to help; don't feel you have to just know it all or be some kind of superwoman. And, above all, don't put pressure on yourself to do anything, especially if this is your first baby. Those of you with toddlers are likely to be far more confident when it comes to taking care of your new baby, but less sure about how to cope with two children. And while I realize doing nothing is not exactly on the cards for you, don't be afraid to still ask for as much help as possible and don't be hard on yourself. If the washing doesn't get done, it's not the end of the world.

A midwife should visit you at home following your delivery to assess both you and your baby. From day ten, the health visitor will see you and take over your care and that of your baby and discuss issues such as immunization schedules for your baby.

Is the Engine Working?

The first thing to say is that from a physiological point of view, childbirth is tough on your body, whether you had a natural or assisted birth.

It is not unusual to experience any of the following after childbirth:

- ❋ **A bloody vaginal discharge (lochia)** Initially this is as heavy as a period and should last for approximately three to four days, after which it will become lighter in colour and volume. It can continue for up to six weeks, gradually turning brown, yellow and then white.
- ❋ **Tearing** If there has been any tearing from giving birth vaginally, there is likely to be some perineal discomfort. It will heal over time, within seven to ten days, and can range from numbness to more acute pain when walking, coughing or sneezing.
- ❋ **Abdominal cramps** These are the after-pains which occur as the uterus continues to contract. Often, these occur when your baby begins to breastfeed and are usually at their most intense in the first forty-eight hours after childbirth, easing over a few days.

❀ **Pain at the site of surgery** If you've had a Caesarean section, there will be pain at the location of the incision, and you need to remember that not only are you recovering from childbirth, but also from major surgery.

❀ **Difficulty urinating** Many women find it difficult to urinate or have a bowel movement in the first twenty-four hours after childbirth. This is often due to anxiety that it will hurt or affect stitches. Acupressure point Kidney 3 may help with urinating.

❀ **Discomfort in the breasts** This is likely to happen as the breasts become engorged on about day three or four and the milk flow changes from rich colostrum to breast milk. This will occur even if you decide not to breastfeed. See Chapter Sixteen for more on breastfeeding and advice on sore breasts and sore or cracked nipples.

❀ **Mood swings** Emotions are intense after childbirth, often swinging between elation and depression. Hormones get in on the act too and are thought to be associated with the 'baby blues' that often come around day three. Even immediately following the birth, many women feel a wave of relief, rather than the 'magic moment' described in so many books and films. I have included a whole section on emotions on p. 317.

The main conditions I look for in the postnatal phase are:

❀ Qi and Blood Deficiency (which can progress to Yin Deficiency)
❀ Blood Stagnation
❀ Coldness and/or Wind penetrating the body
❀ Issues with the Heart.

Blood Stagnation following birth

This is quite common, and I think it is one of those situations that can cause problems for later pregnancies if not addressed properly. Earlier, I talked about the first three days following labour as being a time when the body purges itself. Part of this process is the uterine bleeding that takes place for about ten days after delivery. It is not unusual for there to be discharge and the need to wear a sanitary towel for some weeks after delivery. (Seek advice if you experience any of the symptoms outlined as warning signs on p. 286.)

I quite often see women who have retained products, which we classify as Blood Stagnation, and this needs to be discussed with your healthcare provider. Sometimes, it is not a substantial amount but an energetic imbalance of Blood. If it is not considered serious, acupuncture is an extremely effective way of moving Blood in the uterus, and I'd recommend treatment if you are able to access it. If not, try increasing your intake of foods which move the Blood: aubergine, raspberry-leaf tea, and sipping vinegar in hot water is also a good remedy for clearing blood from the uterus.

Quite often, Blood Stagnation occurs due to Coldness in the uterus. If you feel cold or your tummy is cold to touch, moxa is useful (see p. 295), as is adding some warming foods: ginger, cinnamon, quinoa, jasmine tea, roast chicken with warming herbs, such as sage and thyme, perhaps cooked with a whole garlic in the carcass cavity.

Daverick Leggett recommends tea made of equal parts of cinnamon, ginger and tangerine peel. Place in three cups of water and simmer until the liquid has reduced by half.

Abdominal massage is also helpful, using the essential oils mandarin, orange, bergamot and rose.

Acupressure for after-pains

❀ Spleen 6 is useful to help ease after-pains, which can be quite intense while feeding.

❀ Partner can apply pressure to both legs while baby is feeding.

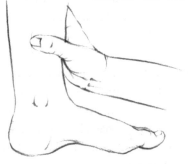

SP 6 IS FOUND FOUR FINGERS' WIDTH ABOVE THE TIP OF THE INSIDE ANKLE BONE IN THE FLESHY DIP BETWEEN THE TWO BONES

HELPS DILATE THE CERVIX AND ESTABLISH LABOUR

YOUR PERINEUM

Unless you had a Caesarean, this area will feel sore and bruised and you might have stitches or small tears that need to heal. Here are some things to try which might help with recovery:

- Keep any stitches clean and dry.
- Pelvic-floor exercises (see p. 299) are helpful for healing.
- Eat plenty of fibre and drink plenty of fluids.
- Soak in a bath with a few drops of lavender oil.
- More raspberry-leaf tea!
- A cold compress of witch hazel can help with bruising and swelling.
- Arnica tablets may reduce soreness from bruising.

Warning signs for possible complications

There are a number of complications to be aware of in the hours and days after birth. If you experience any of the warning signs, always contact your GP or health visitor immediately.

Retained products

If the uterus hasn't expelled all of the placenta or membranes, there is a risk of haemorrhage or the development of an infection. Contact your GP or midwife immediately if you experience any of these symptoms:

- ❀ Bleeding that continues for several hours after the first twelve hours and requires a new sanitary towel pad every hour or more.
- ❀ Bright red and heavy bleeding that continues after four days postpartum.
- ❀ Lochia (vaginal discharge) that has an unpleasant smell – anything different from normal menstrual discharge should be checked out.
- ❀ Large blood clots (bigger than the size of a lemon).
- ❀ No lochia may also indicate retained products.
- ❀ Increasing pain in the abdomen following the initial few days after delivery.

❀ If your temperature rises to 38°C or above for a period longer than twenty-four hours.

Deep-vein thrombosis (DVT)

If you experience pain or tenderness in your calf muscle or a sudden sharp chest pain, these can be signs of a blood clot developing within the deep vein of the leg and, in the case of the sharp chest pain, that the clot may have travelled to the lungs.

Infection of Caesarean scar

Swelling, redness and tenderness around the scar are normal, as is a small amount of clear discharge for a few days. Persistent oozing or pus from the wound are signs you should contact your doctor or midwife.

Effects of Labour on Your Baby

As I said right at the beginning of the book, your baby will inherit her pre-natal Jing from you, and there are many factors that affect her postnatal Jing. You provide the postnatal Jing at this early stage of life through the care you give your baby – both physical and emotional.

Babies that have had a difficult time with delivery, particularly if they have been stuck for a while, often become tense, irritable and frightened. This can be because they have retained some of the compression and forces of the labour. The bones of the head at this time are very soft and mould to the mother's bony confines, which can determine how the central nervous system interacts with the body. The following difficulties can be assessed by an osteopath.

❀ Crying, irritable babies
❀ Feeding
❀ Colic
❀ Sleep disturbances
❀ Head shape
❀ Head banging

- ✿ Teething
- ✿ Bonding with mother

Also, babies cannot manage their own stress; and they are all the more suscep-tible to stress precisely because they cannot rely on themselves to survive. This is why you spend so much time keeping your baby relaxed and fulfilled, in balance. As soon as something, however small, isn't quite right, they let you know!

Recovery from a Caesarean section

If you had a Caesarean section, you have even more reason to take it very easy during the first few weeks after giving birth. For most women, it takes at least six weeks to recover, but this varies for every individual. Here are a few tips to help with recovery:

- ✿ A tiny bit of moving, as in a short wander up the corridor, is help-ful once your doctor gives the go ahead.
- ✿ Don't go up and down stairs too much; create a space where you can feed your baby and chill out for much of the day.
- ✿ Don't drive until you can buckle up without pain and are able to turn to look over your shoulder. Also, contact your insurance company to check what their ruling is on this.
- ✿ If you are feeling a pulling sensation when you move or are heal-ing very slowly, ask your doctor for a referral to a physiotherapist to help with your recovery.
- ✿ Pelvic-floor exercises (see p. 299) are helpful to heal from the inside.
- ✿ Some women experience a feeling that they have been cheated of natural birth, however thrilled and relieved they also feel. Talk to sympathetic friends who won't dismiss your feelings, and if these feelings stay with you, do talk to your doctor (see p. 318 for 'baby blues' and postnatal depression).

LIMA'S STORY

At nearly forty weeks, and measuring forty-three weeks, due to polyhydramnios (excessive amniotic fluid), I was more than ready to give birth, so, when offered a sweep [see p. 233] by the consultant obstetrician, I quickly said yes and went home to see if it worked.

At ten the next morning, I had a show and started having gentle contractions every twenty-five minutes which had built to every eight minutes by lunchtime, when I suggested to my husband that we went out with our daughter, as we were unlikely to get another chance for a while. We went in to hospital at 7 p.m. and were sent home again until I was having contractions at the rate of three every ten minutes. I returned home and had a lovely, peaceful acupuncture session which felt very balancing, and I rested for a few hours until 1 a.m. when I woke up to another, much bigger, show and raced into hospital again.

By 7 a.m., I had dilated to 4cm and the decision was made to break my waters. Things progressed slowly, but at 6.30 p.m. I was told to start pushing at the height of each contraction, and since this was the bit that I had really enjoyed when my daughter was born, I was looking forward to the euphoria of delivery and started pushing hard. I could feel the head moving down the birth canal, but unfortunately that was as far as it got over the next three hours, by which point I was tired and demoralized. The midwife called the doctors, who agreed the baby's shoulders were big and making it impossible for me to deliver vaginally without risking shoulder dystocia. Given the amount of time spent in second stage of labour, it was felt that it would be good to get the baby delivered as soon as possible and that a Caesarean section was the best way to do it. I was wheeled into theatre feeling, frankly, terrified, and as the epidural was turned up very high, I was shaking like a leaf (a standard side effect apparently). My husband was by my side and managed to make me laugh and reassure me by listing everyone we knew who had had a C-section (a surprisingly long list) and, before I knew it, we heard the sound of our son yelling, and I was crying with joy and relief that everything was OK. Nick held him to my face so I could see him and kiss him and he was perfect.

While the C-section was unplanned and scary, I was just grateful that our little boy and me were OK. I kept thinking that if it had been even fifty years ago, we could have had a very different time and may not have survived at all. The joy of having our son safely delivered kept me going through the long process of being sewn back up and dealing with the intense feelings of nausea caused by the levels of anaesthesia and the exhaustion from hard physical work and no rest. I spent a further three days in hospital and, by the time I left, I was able to walk without too much discomfort and felt well and truly ready to go home.

The most difficult bit has been coping with a much longer, harder recovery period than a natural delivery. I am a fairly independent person normally and found the physical restrictions really tough and isolating, as I couldn't drive, and even the buggy was too heavy for me to bounce down the five steps to the pavement, so a walk was impossible unless someone was around to help – all frustrating side effects I had never considered before. The painkillers were pretty effective, but I tried to stop taking them as soon as possible as the side effects were constipation (not funny when you have layers of stitches through your lower tummy) and overdoing things – because I couldn't feel when I stretched too far or bent over too quickly. It also made it harder to give my two-year-old the physical help I was used to giving, like lifting her on to the loo or into her high chair or picking her up if she fell over. My husband had his work cut out looking after all three of us! Six weeks or more of recovering from a C-section is a pain, and not what I would have chosen, but I know that I have years to enjoy being a parent to my lovely, healthy son.

Miso Soup Lima's Way

Serves 2

500ml (18fl oz) water
2 spring onions, finely sliced
half a thumb's length of ginger, sliced
1 red or green chilli
2 tablespoons miso paste (I like white or yellow)
handful of spinach, tenderstem broccoli or finely chopped cabbage
or carrot
1–2 tablespoons edamame beans (I keep a packet of them in the
freezer)

1. Bring the water to the boil with the green parts of the spring onions (reserve the white parts), the ginger and the whole chilli, so they start to impart their flavour.
2. When the water has boiled, strain the spring onions, chilli (reserve this) and ginger, then add the miso paste, stirring gently. Add the edamame beans and whichever vegetables you are using and gently simmer (don't boil, as this can make the miso taste bitter) for 3 minutes or so.
3. Pour into a big bowl and sprinkle with the white parts of the spring onions. I often add the chilli to taste, finely chopped, and, if I have them, a bit of chopped mint, basil and coriander.

Six-week check-up

You will probably arrange to have a postnatal check at around six weeks with your midwife or GP. The checks should cover the physical and emotional aspects of having a new baby and include:

- ❀ any worries about your health
- ❀ whether your perineum or Caesarean scar are healing well
- ❀ a blood-pressure check

❀ checking that your bowel and bladder are working normally

❀ ensuring that, if breastfeeding, there is no engorgement, discomfort or nipple soreness; or, if bottle-feeding, that your breasts have normalized with no residual pain or discomfort

❀ your midwife or GP chatting to you about your mood to check gently for signs of postnatal depression (see p. 318)

❀ any worries you may have about the baby

❀ checking that you are you well supported at home

❀ checking how you are sleeping

❀ a discussion about contraception.

The six-week check-up is really important, but to my mind, how you recover before this check-up is vital, so over the next few pages I will focus on this time and how you can take the best care of yourself possible. After all, I'd say you certainly deserve it.

Nourish the mother to nourish the child

*A person takes the mother as foundation
and the father as shield.*

The Yellow Emperor's Classic of Internal Medicine

Now I wouldn't go so far as to use the phrase 'take to your bed', but rest and recovery are vital after childbirth. Do not underestimate the restorative quality of sleep. It is so important to rest, and sleep when your baby sleeps. In the first few weeks (even months) don't rush around doing 'stuff' when baby is asleep. Use this time to recharge your engine and make sure your milk supply is plentiful. Sleep is especially important if you experienced heavy blood loss during labour. But even with the easiest of labours, you will feel tired and ache for a few days afterwards.

In Chinese medicine, the first three days after childbirth are considered a time of elimination. These three days are followed by thirty days of tonification, when a mother builds up the Blood and Qi – her energy and vitality – lost through pregnancy and birth.

Pregnancy and childbirth leave a woman in a state of imbalance, simply because of the huge reserves of energy needed. This state of weakness relates to an excess of Yin energy, and so, during this month, a new mother needs plenty of warmth and Yang to redress the balance.

The traditional Chinese 'rules' for Doing the Month are not all incredibly practical in this modern day and age, but many are grounded in common sense so that they may be adapted and related to our own lives. Here are my favourites:

❀ Do not go outside for the entire month. I adapt this rule to encourage my patients to rest fully and recover after childbirth, rather than rush back to the outside world.

❀ Do not eat any raw or cold food. It's important for new mothers to stay warm, both on the outside and on the inside. That's why I encourage comforting soups and stews.

❀ Eat chicken and chicken soup. By now, you probably know I could write an entire book on the benefits of chicken soup. Chicken is restoring and warming, we all crave chicken soup when we are ill because it is so nutritious and yet easy to eat.

❀ Do not be blown on by the wind. This sounds a bit strange at first, but relates to the external causes of disease, and suggests that it is best to protect yourself from the outside elements during this vulnerable time, particularly the wind and the cold.

❀ Do not go to other people's homes. Friends will often be sensitive to this in terms of not wanting to pass any germs on to the baby, but in Chinese medicine terms it's for your benefit too.

❀ Do not read or cry. This relates to your emotional vulnerability during the month, as your heart chakra is open during this time, making you extremely sensitive to external emotions. The instruction is a bit crude, but the intent is, again, one of protection for you.

MOTHER WARMING

Josie had lost quite a lot of blood during her twenty-hour labour, and although all had turned out fine in the end and she had delivered a lovely little boy, she was shattered.

Josie felt very cold and shivery and was still bleeding quite heavily. She said she felt weak and slightly dizzy; her midwife had checked her blood pressure, which was slightly low. She felt tearful and was beginning to fret that she would not be able to cope unless she improved. This was only making matters worse.

Five days postpartum, I returned to see Josie and we did some Mother Warming (see p. 295). I showed Paul, Josie's husband, how he could help her by doing this, and I left them with instructions to do it every day. I also left a press needle (see p. 333) in top of Josie's head on the point Du 20.

Josie's mum was staying to help cook and feed Josie while she recovered, so we talked about the sorts of foods that would help Josie. Blood-nourishing foods were a must, due to the blood loss and also warming foods, like ginger, to help bring the warmth and Yang back into Josie's tired body. Ideal dishes were chicken cooked in plenty of ginger, risotto (made with chicken stock) with chestnuts and butternut squash and chicken soup, of course, with plenty of ginger and spring onion.

The Mother Warming helped Josie regain her energy. She stopped bleeding soon after we started and said she felt lifted both energetically and emotionally. She was no longer tearful, and was now able to maintain a constant temperature, instead of sitting shivering while everyone else appeared just right.

These simple methods are often so effective because they help gently to recover the energy. But they require a basic understanding of energy and what the individual needs. Eating salads, trying to do too much or going outside in the cold could have pushed Josie in the wrong direction. It would have been much harder to recover her energies had this been the case. But understanding that she needed warmth and rest was enough to help start her on the road to recovery.

MOXA FOR MOTHER WARMING

Using moxa postnatally is a wonderful restorative treatment that can be done by your partner, friend or whoever is caring for you. Moxa is used to warm the channel that runs on the midline of the body underneath your tummy button to the top of your pubic bone. Whoever is doing this for you will need to follow the instructions for using moxibustion (p. 333), but it is very simple and safe.

There are two types of moxa sticks available. In clinic, I use the original variety, but they tend to be rather smoky and not the best idea for a newborn baby. I would go for the smokeless variety (although they are hard to light, so be patient).

Holding the moxa stick about 2.5cm from the body, start at the tummy button, then slowly trace the midline down towards the top of the pubic bone. Then trace the line back up towards the umbilicus; do this for ten minutes.

If you have had a C-section you should not use this point.

Note: If there are signs of Heat – such as temperature, night fever, looking red in the face, tossing the bed covers off or infection in general – then moxa should not be used..

Postnatal essential oils

Gentle massage using essential oils based in a carrier oil or a few drops added to the bath or a diffuser can be wonderfully comforting and restoring at this time. A good aromatherapist will always talk to you first about how you are feeling on any particular day, to then create an individual blend to suit your mood or how you are physically. I have included here some essential oils for conditions and feelings often experienced by women in the weeks after giving birth.

How to use essential oils
- ❀ For massage: mix thirty drops in 30ml vegetable massage oil
- ❀ In a room diffuser: two to three drops
- ❀ In the bath: four to six drops

Essential oils to treat the Heart
- ❀ Rose Otto is my first oil of choice for the postnatal period. It

is wonderfully uplifting and calming and benefits both mother and baby. I suggest making up a blend of the best-quality rose Otto you can financially justify; mix five drops of essential oil in 10ml base oil (almond oil or virgin olive oil if you are concerned about nut products). Massage this over your body after a morning shower or evening bath.

❀ Rosemary: for feeling cold, lack of enthusiasm and feeling apathetic.

❀ Jasmine: for lack of enthusiasm, apathy and feeling emotional with a lack of joy.

❀ Chamomile: for feeling unable to cope.

❀ Lavender and rose: for feeling anxious and down without energy or joy (the tip of the tongue is normally red).

❀ Cinnamon and camphor: when there is shivering and cold with no energy and anxiety.

❀ Grapefruit: uplifting and energizing, a perky little number that is great for irritable types.

Essential oils for haemorrhoids

Cypress: add two to three drops to a basin of warm water; perch over this with your bottom submerged for soothing relief.

Sweaty Betty

Sweating after childbirth is not considered to be abnormal; indeed, it is part of the body's way of eliminating excess fluid. In Chinese medicine, in the few days following childbirth, the body is still concerned with 'purging'. So sweating would be seen as part of the cleansing process. Some women have retained quite a lot of fluid in the ankles, wrists and even the face; most of this will be lost within days of birth.

If the sweating goes on for more than a few days and leaves you drenched, it would be viewed as an imbalance of Qi and Blood. In clinic, we are usually able to clear this up very quickly with the acupressure points Heart 6 and Kidney 7, but my guess is that these points would not be strong enough through acupressure. If you are able to, it would be worth visiting an acupuncturist and asking them to needle these points (or whatever they felt appropriate); if not, follow the suggestions below. Herbal medicine is also very good here, but you need to work with a herbalist as small traces of herbs will be transmitted to the baby.

Sweating in the day
This is considered a Qi Deficiency and moxa can be used to help build the Qi. Moxa on St 36 is excellent (see p. 112). Rest and eat foods to nourish Qi. Essential oil of rose is helpful too; use a few drops in the bath.

Sweating during the night
This is considered a Yin Deficiency (advanced Blood Deficiency), perhaps through blood loss during labour. Moxa should not be used here, but foods to nourish the Yin will help and taking rest between feeds is vital. Avoid all stimulants, coffee, alcohol, spicy foods or chocolate. Essential oil of rose is an excellent tonic for you – again, use a few drops in the bath. It is very expensive, but you are 'worth it', and you have a big job on your hands and need to keep your strength.

Pains in the joints
Postnatal aches and pains are not very widely talked about. We tend to talk a great deal about labour pain, but women are often surprised when they suffer joint pain in the postnatal period.

Numbness, soreness, a heavy feeling in the limbs and just plain aches and pains are all signs that the Blood needs to be nourished. Remember 'it takes a drop of mother's Blood to make a drop of milk'. If the Blood is weakened from childbirth and breastfeeding, the channels of the body are easily invaded by Cold and Wind. This is why it is so important to wrap up warm after childbirth and not to expose yourself to the elements. I know it sounds terribly old-fashioned, but I see so many problems in clinic that can be traced to the postnatal period.

Consider the following:

❀ If the pains are heavy in nature and you feel sluggish and without energy, including your thought processes and your general powers of concentration, it may be that too much Dampness has penetrated the body. Follow the rules for clearing Dampness (p. 31); and moxa (see p. 295) is also good in this situation.

❀ If the pains are severe and the joints feel stiff, this is Blood Stagnation and it is important to keep the Qi moving around the body so that the Blood does not continue to stagnate. Massage is great for this, and using a blend of essential oils will help to invigorate the Blood in the channels. I recommend ten drops of lavender, five of thyme and ten of eucalyptus diluted in 30ml of almond oil; or simply twenty drops of lavender diluted in 30ml of almond oil.

❀ If the pains move from place to place, this is too much Wind in the body. This is not 'wind' as in 'Who ate all the Brussels sprouts?' but Wind that blows the leaves off a tree. The theory is that when the Blood is weak, then the Wind gets into the body and causes pains that move. This type of pain responds well to warming the body using moxa and to nourishing the Blood.

❀ Blood Deficiency pain is dull and numbing with a tingling sensation. It improves with rest, Blood-nourishing foods and moxa.

Regaining fitness and postnatal exercises

Take it slowly – think of a year plan to get your body back in shape. It will be a different shape and may even be better for all the work you do. Don't attempt any exercise without talking to your doctor or health visitor first, as they will know the exact circumstances of the birth, and what is best for your body's recovery. In general, women who have had a Caesarean are usually advised not to do any strenuous exercise or heavy lifting for the first couple of months. But everyone can practise their pelvic-floor exercises.

First week

Although birth can feel like an exciting time, and the changes are many post-delivery, it is important to rest and take the transition week easy in terms of exercise – as well as everything else.

Pelvic floor

Start gently with pelvic-floor exercises (see p. 206). Doing ten pelvic-floor lifts every time you feed your baby can help you start to see the benefits. Remember as important as it is to lift and squeeze your pelvic floor, it is also important to relax completely between the contractions. A healthy muscle is long and strong.

Abdominals

Start gently by just squeezing on your out breath, and getting a sense of these muscles again. Do this as often as you think about it. Put a sticker on your mobile phone or download the maxosteopaths app (see Resources, p. 344) to set up a regular alarm to help you to remember.

Two to six weeks

Be gentle with yourself and continue to take lots of care during these few weeks. Regaining physical tone varies from mother to mother. Some are back in their normal shape within a few weeks and others take a lot longer. What is important is to respect your body, particularly while breastfeeding, eat a healthy diet and get into the habit of postnatal exercises to help you get back in shape and feel good. We are all unique.

The hospital will routinely give you a sheet of exercises for the first few weeks.

Pelvic floor

You cannot do enough of these. Every hour is good, or building up to four sets of one hundred every day. To do a pelvic-floor exercise well takes concentration. Find quiet and focus to make these exercises count; they will prevent stress incontinence (leaking when laughing, running, coughing) and help you to regain a healthy sex life.

Abdominals

Start with gentle sit-ups:

❀ Lie on your back with your knees bent, lift your bottom gently off the floor and flatten the arch in your back (pelvic tilt).

❀ Tuck your chin into your chest and slowly lift both head and shoulders off the floor using arms as a counterbalance, point your hands to the top of your knees (rolling a pencil up and then down your knees can help focus). Hold this position for five seconds.

❀ Slowly lower yourself to the floor and relax completely.

❀ Repeat three to ten times. If you have no back pain, you can also roll your knees slowly from side to side in this position. This improves your waistline.

Tips for looking after your back and your baby

❀ Keep your head over your pelvis whenever possible, bending your knees to pick your baby up.

❀ Hold your baby centrally with both hands whenever possible to avoid being on one hip for a prolonged length of time.

❀ Use a baby sling to help distribute weight evenly, making sure it provides support for both your baby's bottom and thighs. Don't use for a prolonged length of time.

❀ Put your changing station at waist height (chest of drawers), ensuring you have everything necessary at hand.

❀ As they get older you might want to kneel down over a bed or use the floor, especially as they begin to wriggle.

❀ Kneel down to your child as they get older, inviting them to you, not having to lift them.

❀ Strap your baby into the car seat in the car. This avoids twisting with a heavy weight.

Yoga for postnatal recovery: the first month

Yoga in pregnancy is a very positive investment that pays huge returns in the postnatal period. So many of the practices learnt in pregnancy can be of value in the time of great adjustment to motherhood and to the arrival of your baby.

Use the golden thread breath (see p. 250) as a powerful way to free yourself from the stresses and demands of the labour and birth. Sense how the exhale enables you to let go of the challenges that have gone before, to cleanse yourself of any tensions, and to move forward freely to embrace life with your baby. Sigh, yawn and breathe out tiredness, anxiety and confusion. Consciously breathe in the love, excitement and delight of welcoming a new soul to your family.

Healing and nourishing breath

Take time now to rest and heal; use the healing breath as a tool to ensure that your recovery is happening from the inside out. Every exhalation, gather up the muscles of the pelvic floor and squeeze, drawing them up and inwards, as you encourage the lower-belly muscles to retreat, drawing upwards and inwards. It can take months to get a clear sense of how the pelvic floor is moving after birth, but if you focus your attention with this healing breath, then you bring the capacity to heal and nourish into your pelvic area on every breath. To begin with, there may be only a very tiny response, but even this is beneficial, because you are taking your mental energy and *prana* to the area, encouraging complete healing and nourishing in all the muscles by promoting a positive blood circulation to the tissues of the vagina and the rest of the pelvic floor. Sense that each exhalation brings a loving massage to the organs of the pelvis, drawing in the belly to settle the organs back into place.

It is very common for women who have just given birth to experience stress incontinence and piles or haemorrhoids. Your healing breath can help to strengthen the muscles that close your pelvic sphincters. Practise often, with a free-moving breath, to develop your confidence that these muscles will return to their former glory. It can be a slow process, but the yoga healing breath is a boon. The muscles and tissues have been stretched, opened and moved aside, so the gentle healing encouragement of the yoga squeezes: exhale and lift, over and over again, can be of great benefit at this time. The same gentle action of squeeze and release, squeeze and release, is also very helpful in managing piles, since repeated practice boosts blood flow to the area, speeding healing. Piles can be excruciatingly painful, so it is also very useful to call upon the golden thread breath, especially when defecating, as an effective way to manage pain by exhaling through the intensity.

Pelvic scoops

Restoring the strength of the pelvic-floor muscles is only one small part of the story of postnatal recovery. The pelvic organs depend upon correct posture to ensure their good alignment and resettling into optimal relationship with each other and within the pelvis. So in addition to the healing breath described above, it is valuable to practise pelvic scooping, as a way to realign the pelvis and strengthen the muscles which maintain positive posture. The practice boosts vitality and promotes holistic healing, and has the advantage of being something that is easily done while holding your baby.

The recommended easy hold in the early days is the 'tiger in the tree' hold, in which the baby rests on their belly along your forearm, facing down, with their cheek tucked in close to your elbow. This is a comforting hold for the child, and it keeps your posture balanced.

Stand with feet about hip-width apart and knees bent. As you inhale, allow your tailbone to move out behind you, as if you were sticking your tail up in the air. As you exhale, scoop your imaginary tail through and underneath you, as if you were tucking it between your legs. Keep the breath flowing freely, as you begin to link these two movements together in a continuous circular action that scoops your pelvis forward, alternately lengthening and curving in the lower back. Each exhale, as you tuck the tailbone forward, begin to contract the buttocks, and also the lowest abdominal muscles, between the navel and pubic bones. Sense that the rhythmic scooping, contraction and release of these large muscles builds up a warming and strengthening heat that nourishes your spine and the pelvic organs too. If you keep with the practice, you will discover the heat radiating deep inside the pelvis, healing and nourishing the organs, while the movement undulates up through the spine, freeing the neck and shoulders. It's a magical healing practice!

For more information on Uma Dinsmore-Tuli's books and website, and yoga in pregnancy, please see Resources, p. 339, and Further Reading, p. 347.

Is the Fuel Good?

Diet is an extremely important part of recovering your own energy and well-being after childbirth (remember the saying, 'It takes a drop of mother's blood to make a drop of baby's milk'), while also ensuring a great nutritional start for your baby.

I focus on Qi- and Blood-building foods during this time, including:

❈ oats, rice, potatoes, sweet potatoes, mushrooms, basil, cinnamon, cloves, fennel, ginger, nutmeg, rosemary, thyme and jasmine tea – to nourish Qi

❈ corn, beetroot, dark leafy greens like spinach and kale, apricots, avocados, dates, kidney beans, sesame seeds, eggs, soya milk and red meat – to nourish Blood

❈ goji berries – these are full of vitamins and essential fatty acids;

take about ten to fifteen goji berries and cover in boiling water for three minutes; drink the tea and eat the softened berries for a good pick-me-up.

Food tips for breastfeeding

✿ Pumpkin seeds have been used to help promote lactation.

✿ Breastfeeding consumes a lot of calories. It's important that you are eating enough food, especially food with a good calcium and protein content, such as tofu, spinach, eggs and fish.

✿ Cook foods lightly or slowly to ensure they are more nourishing and easier to digest; raw foods are harder to digest and cold foods are best avoided at this time.

✿ Warm soups and stews are perfect, full of nutrients, comforting and nourishing. Chicken soup is particularly good, so ask your partner to help out. My husband Roger's recipe for chicken noodle soup is below.

Roger's Chicken Noodle Soup

Serves 4

For the stock:

Makes 3.6 litres (6 pints)

1 whole organic/free range uncooked chicken

3.6 litres (6 pints) water

75g (2½oz) ginger, peeled and cut into strips

5 fat garlic cloves (unpeeled)

½ teaspoon salt

2 spring onions

For the soup:

3 pak choi

100g (3½oz) mangetout

100g (3½oz) baby corn

1.2 litres (2 pints) stock (see above)

1–2 red chillies, chopped and deseeded (omit, if you are still having night sweats; some babies don't like chilli breast milk)

2 tablespoons chopped coriander (plus extra for garnish)

4 spring onions, chopped

1 tablespoon light soy sauce

1–2 tablespoons fish sauce (according to taste)

1–2 tablespoons dry sherry or rice wine

1 teaspoon sesame oil

50g (1¾oz) cooked chicken

dried or fresh noodles

1. Place the chicken in a large saucepan. Cover with the water, then add the ginger, garlic and salt. Simmer gently for up to 6 hours, periodically skimming off the fat that rises to the surface with a slotted spoon. If the stock boils it will become cloudy, and the idea is to end up with a clear stock. It may be necessary to add more water during the simmering period to maintain the quantity of liquid.

2. Strain the stock through a fine sieve and keep the best bits of meat for use in the soup. Allow to cool and then freeze for later use.

3. Bring a large pan of water to the boil and add pak choi, mangetout and baby corn. Bring back to the boil and blanch vegetables for 1 minute. Remove from pan and set aside.

4. Heat the stock (do not boil) and add the chillies, coriander, spring onions, soy sauce, fish sauce, sherry or rice wine and sesame oil. Simmer gently for 10 minutes, then add the baby corn. Simmer gently for a further 3 minutes or so, then add the remaining vegetables for a further 2 minutes.

5. Cook the noodles separately. When ready divide them between four soup bowls and pour the soup over the top. Garnish with coriander and serve.

Yin Deficiency

If after childbirth you are suffering from night sweats, irritability, had a heavy loss of Blood and feel slightly feverish then adapt the postnatal diet as follows:

- ❀ Avoid all alcohol, coffee, sugars and heating and pungent spices.
- ❀ Include more adzuki beans, kidney beans, fish in coconut milk, pork, pears, apricots and avocados.
- ❀ When there is anxiety, include barley, celery (cooked), apples, asparagus, mushrooms.

Victoria's Chinese Slow-cooked Pork

This recipe is the perfect tonic to balance Yin and Yang; pork for Yin and the sugar, rice wine and ginger all tonify Yang. Eating rich meat every day isn't so good, but occasionally and eaten with love it is delicious!

Serves 6

1.5 kg (3lb 5oz) pork belly
1.5 litres (2½ pints) chicken stock (see p. 254)
8 Szechuan peppercorns
4 star anise
5 cloves
2 heaped tablespoons brown sugar
1 wine glass Chinese rice wine
1 wine glass soy sauce
1 glug rice wine vinegar

To serve:
plain boiled rice
pak choi or Chinese greens
spring onions, cut lengthways into short, thin strips
thinly sliced ginger
2–3 thinly sliced red chillies

1. Cut the pork belly into large bite-sized pieces and put in a large stock-pot. Cover with the stock and add other ingredients.
2. Bring the stock almost to boiling point. Put the lid on, reduce the heat to its lowest setting and simmer for 2–2½ hours.
3. When the pork is tender, strain the liquid through a sieve. Remove the cloves, Szechuan peppercorns and star anise. Reduce the stock until syrupy.
4. Return the pork to the sauce and turn off the heat. The pork will be happy resting for half an hour.
5. Meanwhile, cook the rice. Serve the pork with rice and steamed pak choi and sprinkle over thinly sliced spring onions, ginger and fresh red chillies.

Yang Deficiency

If after childbirth you are shivery and feel cold with no energy, you need to adapt the postnatal diet as follows:

❀ Avoid cold drinks and raw uncooked foods, champagne, ice cream, yogurt or salads.
❀ Include cooked warm foods that will be more warming in nature: trout, meat (not pork), onions, garlic, ginger, cinnamon, coriander, leeks, radishes, squash, cooked pears with warming spices.

CONGEE[28]

When I describe congee to you as a 'creamy rice soup', you might not immediately want to rush to the kitchen and make a pot. But give it a chance, because I promise it will surprise you – pleasantly. When I told a friend about congee, it reminded her of when she was little and her mother would make her rice pudding if she was ill; it was literally the only thing she could stomach.

Congee is simply rice that is slow cooked in much larger quantities of water than usual. The rice is cooked until it breaks down and turns the liquid thick and creamy. It has a mild, sweet flavour and is incredibly easy on the digestion, so is very nourishing and healing – perfect when you are rebuilding your energy in the weeks after giving birth.

Grains in general are rich in Qi, but our digestion can find it hard to absorb the good nutrition inside them if we don't prepare them properly. Hard grains can be too much for our digestion, especially if it is slightly weakened. Because the stomach can so easily digest the softened grains in congee, however, Stomach Qi increases even as you eat. Often, by eating a little congee, you can actually build your appetite as you eat and feel energized by eating rather than finding it an effort.

Congee is mild and perfect for combining with other flavours, from warm stewed fruit in the morning, to fresh ginger, chicken and sesame oil as a nourishing evening meal.

How to prepare congee

The easiest way to make congee is on the hob. For approximately four servings, rinse 200g (7oz) plain, polished short-, medium- or long-grain white rice (not basmati) and place in a heavy-bottomed saucepan, along with 1.2–2.4 litres (2–4 pints) water (1.2 litres will make a more 'sticky rice' consistency, while 2.4 litres will be quite soupy).

Bring the rice to an easy boil, then reduce to a low simmer for between 30 and 90 minutes, depending on the consistency you prefer. Stir occasionally, to prevent the rice from sticking to the bottom of the pan. The longer you can wait the better.

If you make more than a meal's worth at a time, then reheat just what you need for each meal in a smaller pot. Congee will keep for 2–3 days in the fridge.

If you are making savoury congee, you might want to add some chicken or vegetable stock for a good flavour.

Note: Other grains can also be used in the same way. Oats are sweet, slightly warming and build Blood and Qi, so slow-cooked porridge for breakfast is the perfect start to the day (even better if you soften the oats in water overnight). Spelt grains are strengthening for the Spleen, as well as nourishing for the Blood, and corn builds Blood and Qi, while also helping to build appetite.

Savoury congee recipes

- Chicken congee to build Qi: prepare the congee with chicken broth or stock. Stir-fry chicken in sesame oil and add to the congee in individual bowls, along with thin slices of fresh ginger and spring onions.
- Egg congee to build Blood and Qi: prepare your basic congee with water or chicken stock. Five minutes before serving, crack one egg per person on top of the congee and allow to set before serving. Season with sea salt and pepper.
- Gently sweat onion and grated carrot in olive oil with a little salt and pepper. Add fresh herbs: basil, thyme, rosemary and marjoram (whatever you have) and serve over the congee.

Sweet congee recipes

- Prepare your congee with a few slices of fresh ginger. A few minutes before the end of cooking, add slices of fruit (or stewed fruit), a little honey and a dusting of cinnamon.
- To nourish and cool the Blood: prepare the congee with coconut milk added to the water. Serve with fresh pineapple and banana.

To nourish Blood and Qi

Add any of the following to your congee:

Vegetables
- Swiss chard (Blood)
- Kale (Blood)
- Carrots (Qi)
- Pumpkin (Qi)
- Squash (Qi)
- Watercress (Blood, Qi)
- Shiitake mushrooms (Qi, Blood)
- Reishi mushrooms (Qi, Blood)

Beans
- Adzuki (Blood)
- Lentils (Qi)
- Tempeh (Qi, Blood)

Meat and fish
- Chicken (Qi, Blood)
- Lamb's liver (Blood)
- Pheasant (Qi)
- Turkey (Qi)
- Salmon (Qi, Blood)
- Tuna (Qi, Blood)

Herbs and spices
- Liquorice (Qi)
- Parsley (Blood)
- Sage (Qi)
- Thyme (Qi)

Fruit
- Cherries (Qi, Blood)
- Dates (Qi, Blood)
- Figs (Qi, Blood)
- Papaya (Qi)

Nuts and seeds
- Coconut (Qi, Blood)
- Hazelnuts (Qi, Blood)
- Sunflower seeds (Qi)

Oils and condiments
- Miso (Blood)
- Molasses (Qi, Blood)
- Brown sugar (Qi)

(Nourish me with) Chocolate Beetroot Cake

Beetroot is perfect for nourishing the Blood, as are dates. A slice of this cake will give you a boost – a bit of naughtiness with hidden goodness.

Serves 6

3 medium beetroots
145g (5oz) plain flour
170g (6oz) ground linseeds or flaxseeds
30g (1oz) pure cocoa powder
1 teaspoon bicarbonate of soda
1 teaspoon baking powder
½ teaspoon salt
½ teaspoon ground cinnamon
¼ teaspoon ground allspice
3 extra-large eggs (or 4 small)
200g (7oz) brown sugar
180ml (6fl oz) vegetable or walnut oil
60g (2oz) dates, stoned and chopped
40g (1¼oz) chopped walnuts
For the ganache:
450g (1lb) dark chocolate
240ml (8fl oz) milk

1. Preheat the oven to 180°C/350°F/gas mark 4. Grease and line with parchment paper either a round 23cm (9in) cake tin or a 23 x 13cm (9 x 5in) loaf tin.
2. Remove the stems from the beetroots and boil in their skins for about an hour – remove and set aside to cool.
3. Peel the skins from the beetroots and chop them into chunks – then in a food processor, blitz them again into small pieces, to a coleslaw-type consistency.
4. In a large bowl, sift all the dry ingredients – the flour, ground linseeds, cocoa powder, bicarbonate of soda, baking powder, salt, cinnamon and

allspice. Add the beetroot to the dry ingredients, stirring through, so the pieces are evenly distributed.

5. In another bowl whisk the eggs lightly, and add the sugar and oil. Add this mixture to the dry ingredients, lightly stirring to combine, then stir in the dates and walnuts. Pour the mixture into the cake tin.

6. Bake in the preheated oven for 45 minutes, then lower the heat to 160°C/325F/gas mark 3 and bake for a further 20–25 minutes. Test to see if it's ready by inserting a knife in the middle – if it comes out clean it is ready. Remove the cake from the oven and turn out on to a wire rack. Leave to cool.

7. To make the ganache, melt the chocolate very carefully over a low heat, using a double boiler (a heatproof bowl set over a saucepan of nearly boiling water), while stirring with a wooden spoon. When it is all melted, slowly begin pouring in small amounts of the milk, while continuously stirring. Keep going until all the milk is incorporated into the chocolate – it should be the consistency of double cream, or a little thicker. Remove from the heat and put in the fridge to cool and thicken for at least a couple of hours. (You can do this the day before and leave it overnight – or a couple of hours before making the cake.)

8. When the cake has cooled completely, if you are making the round sandwich version, use a large serrated knife and carefully slice into 2 halves horizontally; if you are making the loaf version, leave whole. Put the cake on a serving plate and spread the ganache, with a palate knife or spoon, either in between the two layers of the round cake, putting the remainder on top, or over the top and sides of the loaf cake.

9. Serve with green tea for an antioxidant-packed dessert that is so rich and delicious you won't even think about how good it is for you!

THREE WAYS WITH ADZUKI BEANS

Adzuki beans are a traditional remedy for improving breast-milk production. Soaked overnight and boiled until soft, they can be used in a number of ways and can be eaten as either a sweet or savoury dish. In *The Baby-Making Bible*, I recommend adzuki beans for those who are too Damp, as they are fantastic at nourishing the digestive system and getting rid of excess Damp. These sorts of patients may suffer from a sluggish digestion, with poor metabolism and a feeling of heavy limbs. They may have a thought process that tends towards rumination and often lack the ability to focus and concentrate on anything.

Sweet Adzuki Bean Porridge

There are a couple of ways to prepare the beans for cooking – either soaking them overnight or parboiling them. Soaked overnight, the beans' texture will be mushy, while parboiling them will result in whole beans cooked in syrup.

Makes 1 bowl

100g (3½oz) adzuki beans
450ml (15fl oz) water
1 strip tangerine or orange peel (optional)
½ teaspoon ground allspice
¼ teaspoon ground cardamom
¼ teaspoon ground cinnamon
2 tablespoons agave syrup
pinch of sea salt

1. If the beans were soaked overnight, bring all the ingredients (except the salt) to the boil, then simmer over low heat for 40–45 minutes. If the beans were not soaked, cover them with a generous amount of water, filling the saucepan to around 5cm above the level of the beans. Bring to the boil for a few minutes. Drain and rinse the beans and discard the cooking water.

Bring all the ingredients (except the salt) to the boil, then simmer over low heat for 60–90 minutes. During cooking, check to see if you need to add more water – eventually the liquid should be a syrupy consistency.

2. For both methods, add the pinch of salt and more agave syrup to taste. Remove the orange or tangerine peel and enjoy with a cup of nettle tea.

Adzuki Bean Salsa

Makes about 4 servings
230g (8oz) adzuki beans
2 large, firm tomatoes
1 small green or red chilli, deseeded and finely chopped
1 medium red onion, finely chopped
1 small bunch coriander, finely chopped
extra-virgin olive oil
¼ teaspoon cayenne pepper (optional)
juice of 2–4 limes, depending on juiciness
salt and pepper to taste

1. Soak adzuki beans overnight in water. Drain and simmer in water for 1 hour. (If you want to make the same day, boil the beans for 2 minutes, then turn off the heat and let them sit for an hour. Drain and replace the cooking liquid with water, bring to the boil, then simmer for 1–1½ hours.)

2. To peel the tomatoes, score the skin with a sharp knife from the stem all the way round – as if cutting into quarters, but not cutting into the flesh. Submerge in boiling water for a couple of minutes, until the edges of the skins curl up and you are able to peel them off easily. Remove the core and the seeds and dice the flesh into 1cm (½in) pieces.

3. Drain the beans and in a serving bowl, combine all the ingredients, adding olive oil and salt and pepper to taste. Serve at room temperature with cold meats and potatoes.

Chicken Minestrone with Adzuki Beans

This is a quick and easy version of chicken soup that can be made when you don't have much time. It can also be made without the chicken as a vegetarian option. The red adzuki beans will turn the outside of the chicken pieces a deep pinkish purple while cooking.

Makes 4 large bowls (or 8 small ones)

200g (7oz) adzuki beans, soaked overnight
8 chicken thighs, skinless and boneless
olive oil
8 large or 12 small garlic cloves, peeled and halved or crushed with
    the back of a knife
2 onions, sliced
125g (4½oz) peas
115g (4oz) green beans
3 small carrots, chopped
75g (2½oz) kale, rinsed and chopped
3 bay leaves
½ teaspoon ground turmeric
½ teaspoon ground allspice
½ teaspoon cayenne pepper
2 teaspoons dried rosemary
2 teaspoons dried thyme
1½ teaspoons dried basil
1½ teaspoons dried oregano
2 teaspoons sea salt (less if using stock or bouillon – add to taste)
1.5 litres (2½ pints) chicken stock, chicken or vegetable bouillon or water
salt and pepper

1. Drain and rinse the adzuki beans and set aside.
2. Slice the chicken thighs into large chunks – 2 or 3 per thigh.
3. Pour 2–3 glugs of olive oil into a large stockpot on high heat. Add the chicken pieces, so that each piece touches the bottom of the pot when

the oil is hot – to sear the meat. After a minute or two turn each piece with tongs, letting them sear on the other side. Take off the heat, remove the chicken pieces from the pot and set aside.

4. Returning the pot to the heat, add the garlic and onions and sauté for a couple of minutes, then add the peas, green beans, carrots and kale, with some more olive oil if needed.

5. Add all the herbs, spices and salt, stirring to lightly sauté while still on a high heat.

6. Add the water or stock, followed by the adzuki beans and bring to the boil with the lid on. After 5 minutes or so, add the chicken pieces and any liquid with them. Bring to the boil again and then simmer for 40 minutes with the lid on.

7. Remove the lid and increase the heat to reduce the liquid, for another 10–20 minutes, depending on how thick you want the soup to be. Add salt and pepper to taste and serve with toasted bruschetta or crostini.

Is the Mind on Board?

In Chinese medicine, we consider your Heart chakra to be open after child-birth. This makes sense as it is a time of bonding and nurturing for this brand new person who depends entirely on you. It also means that many women experience bittersweet feelings during the weeks after giving birth. There are times of elation and intense love, but also new mothers may experience a dip in their emotions or feel more tearful. And, for some reason, this is often on or around day three after having their baby.

Baby Massage by Anna Cannon

After the first four to six weeks – when you and your baby are feeling more like a functioning unit, you are feeling a little less tired, your breasts are comfortable and you feel you have recovered from the birth somewhat – it may be that you are ready to think about going out and about into the big world with your baby. When your baby is around six weeks old, it is a great idea to venture out to some groups for new mums. One group that is particularly advantageous for both mother and child is Baby Massage. Ask your midwife or health visitor about groups in your area.

Baby Massage is fundamentally about communicating love through nurturing touch. It is very relaxing for you and your baby and can help with bonding and preventing postnatal depression. It can help you to understand your baby better and enhance your relationship. For your baby, it can help with issues such as colic, difficulty sleeping and crying. Your baby's muscle development and immune system may benefit and, best of all, it can be practised easily every day for just a few minutes.

Baby hand massage

A tip while breastfeeding is to give your baby a hand massage. I remember my daughters screwing up their fists into tight little balls while furiously trying to feed. Sometimes, I would find little bits of fluff hidden inside their tightly clenched fists. I always thought that it must put a great deal of tension into their digestive systems, so I used my Chinese medicine knowledge of paediatric massage and began to give hand massage while feeding.

- ❀ Using your thumb, gently encourage your baby to relax and open their hand to reveal their palm.
- ❀ Trace a gentle circle on their palm with your thumb using circular movements. I think this works best with your right hand and their left, or their left and your right. Do this slowly and until your baby surrenders and the palm begins to open out.
- ❀ Now massage each finger, one by one, uncurling them as you go. Give the tip of each finger the gentlest of squeezes before you move on to the next one. Once you have massaged each digit, finish the sequence by very gently squeezing your palm to their palm. Remember to use the gentlest touch.

Heart protector

Mothers who are themselves under stress are likely to have more difficulty in regulating their babies well.

Sue Gerhardt, Why Love Matters[29]

I always tell my new mums that they need to look after and protect their Heart (emotions); postbirth the Heart is very vulnerable, and being exposed to sad or shocking images or events can have a detrimental effect.

As a practitioner, I always view the mother and baby as a single unit. By this I mean that their emotions and physical symptoms are as one, intermingled with each other. If the baby is very distressed and crying a great deal, for example, I will check the mother's mood and how she is coping. Equally, a crying, distressed baby is likely to impact on the emotions of even the most confident mother. In Chinese medicine, one of our main principles when giving treatment is, 'Treat the mother, treat the child.' I think this is very powerful; all too often, the baby's needs are addressed without giving due care and attention to the mother, who is, of course, the main caregiver. Happy mother will equal happy baby in many cases.

I remember the terrible events of 9/11 – horrific images of the Twin Towers falling down and the thousands of people who lost their lives in such appalling circumstances. At this time, I remember conversations with new mums and mums-to-be about how they felt traumatized by the images they had seen, yet how, at the same time, many felt compelled to watch them (some obsessively, and while breastfeeding their babies). For many women about to become mothers for the first time, these images were one step too far. On the one hand, the women were bringing new life into the world and experiencing the enormous sense of joy that that brings; but on the other hand, they were asking themselves serious questions about the kind of world they were bringing their child into.

The opposite of joy is feelings of sadness and seriousness. Watching and dwelling on things of a serious nature can damage the Heart energy and make us susceptible to depression. Some of the advice I gave mothers at this time involved not looking at these sad and terrible images. For those who had become fixated on watching them, I advised them to set time aside every day to sing to their baby and to watch and speak about light and simple things. This may sound crazy, but it is effective and there is plenty of time in life to be more serious. Obviously, the events of 9/11 were extreme, and it is always important that we all sit up and pay attention to the suffering of others. But the job of a new mother is to focus on life on a smaller but no-less-important scale – caring for herself and her baby.

Try not to let too many outside influences in – a challenge in itself in these times. Too much information from relatives, friends, the internet and the media can be stressful and create conflicts, the last thing you need. The longer you can cocoon yourself and shut out the rest of the world, the more able you will be to find your feet and to discover how you wish to raise your child, with your own innate skill and knowledge.

Postnatal depression (PND)

Feelings of elation contrasting with times when you feel a little low or lacking in confidence are all normal, but I will still give you some advice you can try on the days you experience a dip (see Tapping, p. 319). However, postnatal depression is something that needs to be taken very seriously, so if you experience low feelings which last for longer than a few days at a time, you should talk things through with your doctor.

Warning signs of postnatal depression
- ❈ Feeling low for long periods of time – a week or more
- ❈ Tearfulness
- ❈ Irritability
- ❈ Panic attacks
- ❈ Lack of motivation or interest
- ❈ Lack of concentration
- ❈ Feelings of loneliness, guilt or inadequacy
- ❈ Feeling unable to cope
- ❈ Finding it difficult to sleep, even though very tired
- ❈ Headaches or stomach aches as a result of tension

Many of the problems with mood and depression that I see in clinic have their roots in Blood Deficiency that has been allowed to continue unchecked. This is why I repeat myself so much from an early stage in pregnancy, as prevention is always better than cure. Working right up until the time of delivery and returning to normal activities too quickly does not help in the long run. It's important to support new mothers so that they can stay well.

Tapping for baby blues

For some women, the fear of baby blues far outweighs the reality of the feelings, and many, many people experience this hormonal dip without going on to develop full postnatal depression. The women who worry about it tend to be those with a history of depression and, for them, the 'baby blues' can be a very frightening thing to anticipate. Tap in advance to clear these fears:

- ❀ 'Even though I am scared of feeling depressed, I deeply and completely love and accept myself.'
- ❀ 'Even though I am frightened of getting the baby blues, I deeply and completely love and accept myself.'

When women do experience this dip in mood a few days after giving birth, the most important thing they can do is actually to recognize it. Often, they are so exhausted and overwhelmed by the birth and looking after their newborn baby that all clear thinking is lost. It is important to know that this is a normal biological process, and it will pass. Sometimes, women will feel that they are not coping, that they are failures. Many 'shoulds' appear at this time. The following tapping protocols may be useful, but, as ever, it is important to adapt them to suit the individual feelings.

- ❀ 'Even though I am not coping, I deeply and completely love and accept myself.'
- ❀ 'Even though I can't stop crying, I deeply and completely love and accept myself.'
- ❀ 'Even though I should be happy, I deeply and completely love and accept myself.'
- ❀ 'Even though I feel so low, I deeply and completely love and accept myself.'
- ❀ 'Even though I feel like a failure, I deeply and completely love and accept myself.'

Comparing ourselves to others

A truly human trait is the desire to compare ourselves to others. We are all, by our nature and our upbringing, pretty competitive beings. It's understandable that as new mums we are desperate to show we can cope, and often, this might mean women either conceal their true feelings or charge back into the real world too quickly, wanting to be seen as exactly the same woman who left work just a short time before.

Feelings of anxiety are completely natural, but if left, they can stagnate and generate a negative cycle of thoughts. They might even create anger and resentment that comes out in bursts or gets pushed inside. Seeing women letting go of this sense of competition in my practice is very rewarding because it can be life-changing for them.

So don't worry if other mums in your group or circle of friends are creating a routine for their babies, but you don't feel ready to start thinking about this. Don't think negatively about yourself if you snap at your older children because you're exhausted – do think about it, but in more constructive terms than negative comparisons with perfection.

I believe the tradition of taking it easy for a month and all that goes with that is well worth paying attention to. I see so many women who rush back to 'normal' but, of course, it's not really normal at all, as things have been changed for ever and nothing will be as it was before. It's important to realize how much your life has changed, and to spend some time simply being with your baby. You will never have this time again, so I really encourage you to make the best of it and to lay sound foundations for the many years to come. A woman's health can change for better or worse at this time, so make sure you use it wisely. It will give you and your baby a fantastic start from which to grow.

chapter sixteen
BREASTFEEDING

by Anna Cannon

Breastfeeding is a symbiotic process; that is to say that mother and child are mutually reliant on each other for its continuation. It is a wonderful process that in many ways encapsulates what it means to be a woman. It crosses countries, cultures and class.

For both you and your baby, some time might be needed to get the hang of breastfeeding. Each mother's milk is different; it will vary depending on the time of day, the age of your baby and to a certain extent your diet. You may notice that sometimes your baby wants to feed from both breasts until you feel there's no milk left (but there *always* is by the way – your baby only ever takes about two thirds of available milk), wherea other times he may want just a little or a snack from one side. It doesn't mean he is ill or doesn't like your milk – it's just a case of, 'That's all I want at the moment, Mum.' The important thing is to listen and watch for your baby's cues. As time passes, you will do this subconsciously and become more confident about understanding your baby, but in the early days, it may feel like there is no particular pattern to your baby's feeding. That's completely normal, so just go with the flow!

Breastfeeding can even help with the weaning process. Your baby gets accustomed to family foods and flavours through your milk. Sometimes, if you eat a lot of orange foods, such as carrots, your milk may have a tinge to it, or it can be garlicky or gingery. All this leads to variety, which is always good.

Don't forget though, that breastfeeding may be a natural activity but that doesn't mean it is always easy. Sometimes, there are obstacles that are just too difficult to scramble over in getting breastfeeding established. If you find that despite seeking advice from your lactation consultant or healthcare professional, you are still having difficulties, it is OK to decide it's not working for you and your baby. The most important element is your relationship with your baby and your happiness and enjoyment.

Getting Started

Although your breasts need no preparation when you are pregnant (nature takes care of that) it is helpful to think about what breastfeeding will be like for you. If you can, try to go along to a breastfeeding workshop in your local area (the easiest way to find one is to look online or ask your health visitor) or speak to your local lactation consultant, so you can learn some of the basics, which is of great help for the very early days.

Uninterrupted skin-to-skin contact between you and your baby as soon as she is born is important for helping to establish breastfeeding. This means wherever possible for your baby to be put on your tummy or chest immediately after birth. The effect this has is profound. Your baby feels safe and secure in your arms, comforted after the trauma of birth, warmed by your skin to prevent her from getting cold and, amazingly, after a few minutes she may even wriggle up to your breast and latch on all by herself.

If you have had a Caesarean, don't worry, as your baby can still cuddle up to you soon after the birth. If, for any reason, you are unwell and unable to do skin-to-skin contact, your partner and baby can do it together. Ensure your midwife knows about your wishes, and she will be happy to help baby slip under your partner's T-shirt.

KANGAROO CARE

The principles of kangaroo care – where you hold your baby skin-to-skin as much as possible – are very simple, and research has shown huge benefits to unwell and premature babies.

When babies are kept next to their mother's skin they thrive. They are able to maintain their temperature better, as the mother's breast temperature goes up and down depending on the baby's. They have a lower heart rate and their breathing is regulated by their mothers. They use fewer calories and have reduced levels of stress. Babies who experience kangaroo care grow at a faster rate and despite the problems of being premature or unwell, the important bonding process is interrupted far less.

If your baby is unwell and separation is necessary, it is important to touch your baby as often as possible. This may be a reassuring stroke of her back or a little bit of touch relaxation or baby massage. And, if at all possible, speak to the paediatricians and midwives involved in your baby's care about kangaroo care (see box).

Soon after birth

For the first three days or so after your baby is born, you have colostrum in your breasts. This is a wonderful food, extremely nutritious, containing everything your baby needs. Colostrum is rich in many nutrients, including vital antibodies to protect your baby from infections. It also encourages your baby to pass meconium which can contribute to jaundice if it remains in their body. It is also thought that the hormone oxytocin that is so helpful during labour is circulated between you and your baby during breastfeeding. This hormone is likely to leave both of you feeling slightly sedated and satisfied after breastfeeding.

It is a fallacy that babies need large amounts of food to help them settle and sleep. On the first day of life your baby's stomach is the size of a small marble and can hold only about 5–7ml. On the third day, it is about the size of a large marble and can hold about 22–27ml. On days seven to ten their stomach is about the size of a ping-pong ball and can hold 30–60ml. Your newborn baby will generally want to feed about eight to twelve times in twenty-four hours. Try not to be too concerned about routine and time limits though. Remember that when you were pregnant your baby was being fed constantly via the umbilical cord. Now she is out, she has to learn to get used to digesting food and taking food in a different way and this can understandably take some time.

Breastfeeding works in such a way that the more often your baby goes to your breast, the more milk you will make. Given these quantities, it is easy to see that a baby needs to feed little and often on the colostrum in the early days and until your milk 'comes in'. This is usually around day three, though it may be later if you have had a very long labour, a Caesarean or if you are diabetic.

Acupressure for breastfeeding

Apply pressure to Gb 34 prior to feeding to help establish the milk let-down reflex.

Very calming if the woman feels anxious, Gb 34 is located a finger's breadth outside the point St 36, below and in front of the bone (see p. 112 for an illustration of St 36).

Learning to Feed Comfortably

Being comfortable and learning how to hold your baby takes some practice initially. It is worth having a go with a doll while you are pregnant at either your antenatal group or a breastfeeding workshop, or you could speak to your midwife.

Getting the latch right is a fundamental step to pain-free and efficient breastfeeding. Ask your midwife to help you as it can be difficult to get it right at first. There is a variety of positions you can try, including lying down, which is a wonderful one to master especially for night time. The cradle position is likely to be the first and most common one you will use.

Cradle position

If you are feeding from your left breast, your baby should be held comfortably in your right arm. Her body should be in a nice straight line, with her head and neck aligned with the rest of her body. (Tummy should be to Mummy.) In this position, your baby is not twisted or stretched. Imagine how difficult it would be to drink if your chin was over your shoulder! Your baby's head should be supported in the 'V' shape of your right thumb and forefinger enabling her to extend her head back to open her mouth wide. Don't be tempted to push your baby's head to your breast. She won't like that. Her nose should be opposite your nipple and you need to think about aiming your nipple right to the back of her throat. Babies don't always latch on straight away; sometimes they like to sniff and just 'hang out' there a bit first. You may want to express a little bit of milk or colostrum to encourage her. When she is ready she will open her mouth. Wait until she really opens wide and almost exaggerate the amount of breast you are guiding into her mouth. She should have a good amount of areola in her mouth and her chin should be slightly indenting the underside of your breast though this will be difficult for you to see. Her cheeks should be full and rounded, her lips curled out. There should be no clicking or sucking sounds. Most importantly it shouldn't hurt.

Let your baby feed for as long as she wants to. This way she will get a balanced feed. Breastfeeding is most successful with unrestricted feeding. With proper attachment, your baby will feed efficiently and come off your breast herself when she has had enough. Remember, breastfeeding is about supply and demand. Your baby demands to her needs and your breasts supply exactly what she needs. This is why it is important not to supplement with formula or to give dummies. If your baby isn't suckling at the breast in an unrestricted way, your breasts are unable to make the required amount of milk.

You will know by your baby's behaviour if you need to offer her the second breast once she has finished on the first. Sometimes, she may want both breasts, sometimes one. When she has finished, she will fall off the breast in a satisfied stupor.

MOBILE PHONES

I worry about the use of mobile phones while feeding your baby as we don't yet have a full picture of the effect of long-term exposure. Probably, the danger to a brain protected by a nice thick fully formed skull is negligible, but I do worry about mobile phones being so close to newborn babies. And there's also the issue of using this time to focus and bond with your baby. If you are distracted by talking or texting on the phone, your baby will know that your attention is elsewhere and may feel insecure. Use this time to simply look into your baby's eyes and rest.

Tray-baked Ratatouille with Brown Rice

This recipe is really simple and tasty and doesn't require a great deal of effort (or washing up at the end, which is good when you're tired after a day feeding and looking after your baby). The ratatouille is also good served with grilled chicken breast or lamb chops for an extra protein kick.

Serves 2 hungry people (one of whom is breastfeeding!)

1 aubergine

1 red pepper

1 red onion

2 bay leaves

4 garlic cloves

1 sprig rosemary

extra-virgin olive oil

red wine vinegar

sea salt and freshly ground pepper

4 or 5 fresh organic tomatoes (or, preferably, 12–15 organic cherry
   tomatoes)

1. Preheat oven to 200°C/400°F/gas mark 4.
2. Slice the aubergine into 2cm (¾in) chunks and chop the pepper into similar-sized pieces. Slice the red onion into wedges. Put all the vegetables into a roasting tray with the rosemary, bay leaves, garlic (skinned, left whole and bashed with a pestle), plenty of olive oil, a splash of red wine vinegar, sea salt and freshly ground pepper and the tomatoes.
3. Toss all the vegetables together and roast for 30 minutes. Check and toss again, then roast for a further 10 minutes, until the vegetables are soft and the onion slightly caramelized.
4. Serve with brown rice and crème fraîche or plain yogurt mixed with lemon juice and chopped fresh parsley.

Common Problems

In Chinese medicine, there are generally two explanations for breastfeeding problems: Qi and Blood Deficiency or Liver Qi Stagnation.

Qi and Blood Deficiency

You feel tired, pale and have no appetite. Causes might be exhaustion, blood loss during labour, a prolonged labour or working right up until labour.

- ✤ Rest is essential.
- ✤ Follow the diet in this chapter to nourish Qi and Blood.

Liver Qi Stagnation

You have hard, painful breasts. You may be irritable and feeling anxious. This picture has far more emotional symptoms and is normally born of anxiety or depression.

- ✤ It is important to get good advice and support (just don't ask too many people!).
- ✤ Try a few drops of grapefruit essential oil in the bath.
- ✤ Acupressure: Ln 3 Si 1 Gb 21 massage Ren 17.

Sore and cracked nipples

The most common problem is sore and cracked nipples. This is generally usually due to an incorrect latch, where the baby is just feeding on the nipple and not having her mouth open enough. This is easily rectified with support from your midwife or lactation consultant, but if you follow the guidelines on p. 324, you should have no pain. Breastfeeding initially may feel a bit strange and uncomfortable until you become more used to it, but it should never hurt and should certainly not become something that you dread.

A mixture of two parts almond oil and one part wheatgerm oil is a good treatment if cracked nipples do occur.

Engorgement

Engorgement is a natural process that happens to all women after they have had their baby, whether they breastfeed or not, as it is hormonally driven. About two to six days after birth, your milk will 'come in'. This means that your breasts will become very full with milk. They will also feel tender, heavy and taut. Sometimes, the swelling can extend to your armpits as breast tissue is found there too. It is a temporary condition, due to an increased blood flow to the breasts, as well as all the extra milk, and it will settle down once your breasts have become accustomed to your baby's demands, usually over two to four days, though this does vary.

You can minimize engorgement by ensuring that your baby is well positioned at the breast and that the latch is good. It will also help if you feed your baby very regularly, eight to twelve times in twenty-four hours. You should also give your baby unrestricted breast feeds. If your baby is unwell or not able to feed this frequently, express your milk a similar number of times using a good breast pump.

It is also common when your milk 'comes in' to feel unwell. You are likely to feel hot, feverish, weak and a bit like you have flu. These symptoms do not last long but look after yourself and get lots of rest in bed. If you do have a temperature it is a good idea to take some paracetamol as prescribed.

The following should help you to find some considerable relief:

- ❀ Breastfeed frequently using both breasts.
- ❀ Try gentle breast massage during feeding.
- ❀ Apply cold flannels to breasts between feeds.
- ❀ Place hot flannels on your breasts just before feeding, for five minutes or so.
- ❀ Sit in a hot bath or shower.
- ❀ Put cabbage leaves in your bra.
- ❀ Wear a good-fitting, supportive bra.
- ❀ Sometimes when your breasts are very full your baby may find it difficult to latch on. If this is the case, you may need to hand express a little milk to soften your breasts to enable your baby to latch on adequately.

Blocked ducts and mastitis

If you develop a hard, painful lump in your breast, this is likely to be a blocked duct. If a section of your breast becomes red, sore, hard and painful, then more than one duct is involved and you may have developed mastitis, where the breast is not being drained properly and milk is becoming stagnant. If you think you may have a blocked duct or mastitis you need to speak to your lactation consultant, midwife or GP.

There isn't much worse than the soreness of a blocked duct that can lead or already has led to mastitis. This can really test your commitment to breast-feeding, and putting your baby to the breast is likely to be the last thing you feel like doing. By acting fast, using the following three simple steps, you can help to relieve yourself of the symptoms of a blocked duct or mastitis:

- ❁ Apply heat (using a hot flannel, hot-water bottle or hot shower) to the affected breast.
- ❁ Go to bed with your baby if you can. Rest is very important.
- ❁ Breastfeed your baby frequently on the affected side.

Sometimes, mastitis can be caused by bacteria entering the breast due to cracked or sore nipples, so correct attachment is vital. Again, get your midwife or lactation consultant to check if you are unsure. It is most likely that you will need to have a course of antibiotics if you develop mastitis, but also try the following:

- ❁ Get to an acupuncturist as soon as possible.
- ❁ Concentrating on the affected area, gently massage your fingers around it in a circular pattern to enhance drainage.
- ❁ It is important to continue feeding as much as possible on the affected side to drain the breast. Sometimes, mastitis makes your milk taste a bit salty so your baby may not be keen to feed as enthusiastically as before (though this milk is not bad for your baby to drink). If this is the case, it is important that you express your milk using either a good breast pump or hand expressing as regularly as your baby would feed. Don't forget that you need to be emptying your breast regularly throughout the night as well. As a rule this means every two to three hours.

❀ You will find that changing the position in which your baby is latched on will help too. Try pointing your baby's chin to the affected area to aid drainage. This may mean some unusual positions for you and your baby, such as leaning over your baby and letting your breast hang loose or feeding in a semi-recumbent position with your baby over your shoulder. Don't be worried about trying new positions, it will all help.

❀ Often, mastitis is caused by stress and overtiredness which is understandable with a new baby, but try to minimize your stress as much as possible. Let people help if they are offering. Family, friends and neighbours can really help while you rest. It is not uncommon for mastitis to develop if you have been more busy than usual, so try to reduce your workload with a young baby.

❀ Make sure you have a well-fitting bra as one that is too tight can contribute to you developing mastitis.

❀ Use cabbage leaves over your breast, they really help to cool them down.

❀ Massage under the arm and around the breast to move the stuck Qi.

❀ Use a warmed wheat pack before and after feeding.

afterword
BECOMING A MOTHER

I consider myself extremely lucky to have an amazing midwife as my sister-in-law. I also had my children at a time when I was starting out as a practitioner and had all my Chinese medicine and complementary therapies to support me. I had my first daughter Lily in hospital in water, and my second daughter Violet in my bedroom at home. Both girls were delivered by Anna (my sister-in-law); both births were easy and even enjoyable. It took guts to have a home birth and not everyone supported my decision.

Of course, not many people are spared at least some difficulty along the way and it took four pregnancies to have my two girls. This is nothing compared to some of my amazing patients who have put themselves through untold discomfort and heartache to have their babies. I expect every one of those women would tell you it was worth it though.

Becoming a mother is a challenging yet incredible part of any woman's life. It is hard – no one can or should deny that – and I think you are really put to the test. But I wonder if this is for a reason. It is a time of both joy and heartache, full of contradictions as the pendulum swings from one extreme to the other.

For all the joy and excitement you feel, you may wonder if you will cope – with the pain of labour, first of all, but more importantly, with being a mother. On the whole, people do cope and it is what creates that strong bond between humans and their children. No other species invests quite so much time and energy in its offspring as human beings, which is probably why it is relatively hard to conceive, then give birth to them.

I hope that along your journey, you will find the right people to support you through your pregnancy, be they midwives or friends and family who have had babies themselves. There are many good organizations out there to support you too. It's a bit of a balancing act, as you need to be patient and take advice, but you also need to find your own way.

I think it is true of many people that they tend to look to others for everything. This seems to be particularly true when it comes to health. So many of us have lost faith in our own ability to judge, handing our health over to others at the drop of a hat, when really many of the things we worry about could be sorted out simply and without intervention. At the other end of the scale are those who don't ask for help at all, thus endangering their health. Again, there is a balance to be struck, and I hope I have gone some way to teaching that in this book.

I hope that you will begin to trust your intuition and to value common sense. On the one hand, this is a book based on the principles of Chinese medicine, but there are also so many ideas which are just plain common sense. You would be amazed at the brilliant women I have seen over the years who have forgotten the importance of common sense and intuition. But the funny thing about these values is that when encouraged, slowly but surely, they come alive in people. The more you focus on and use your instincts, the stronger they grow and the more confident you become. There is no better time to practise this than now.

I believe there are things that mothers know and do that go beyond the scope of any book or expert telling them 'how to do it'. Having said that, in writing this book, I am guilty of giving you advice. But the reason I feel the need to do this is because, mostly, we have become a generation of adults who seem to have forgotten how to trust our own instincts and who rely instead on books, the internet and the experts to tell us how it's all done. What I am hoping to achieve through this book is to reconnect you to the mother in you – the one who knows what is best for her child; yes, better than me or anyone else.

Becoming a mother was the time in my life when I began to listen to myself and to make my mark on the world; I urge you to do the same.

appendix

Moxibustion and Warming Techniques

In moxibustion, a herbal stick (moxa) is lit and held over acupuncture points or areas of the body in order to warm and activate them. In clinic, I often put moxa directly on to the needle, which is known as 'hot-needle technique'. I also give patients a 'Womb Warmer' to use at home – a small heat pad that can be placed on the lower abdomen and used again and again. (See Resources, p. 339 for information on moxibustion equipment suppliers.)

The techniques are used to warm the body in the case of Cold, Cold/ Damp and Yang Deficient, especially when the lower abdomen is cold to touch.

How to use moxa

I recommend that you visit a practitioner for an introductory session to using moxa. Here are tips you can then use at home:

- ❀ You can buy a traditional or a smokeless variety in the form of a cigar-like stick from Chinese medicine shops. I prefer the traditional, but they are extremely smoky, so if you do go for this option, you may need to use it with the windows open.
- ❀ Before using moxa, you will need to prepare the following: a cigarette lighter or matches, a small ashtray to tap the ash into, a small towel to protect any fabric near where you are using the stick and a glass screw-top jar in which to put out the moxa stick at the end of the treatment.
- ❀ Light one end of the moxa stick. Hold the lit end 2–3cm from the back of your hand and feel the warmth.
- ❀ Hold the lit end of the stick over the area to be treated. Always keep it 2–3cm away from you and never make direct contact with the skin.

- ❀ Acupuncture points can be warmed with the moxa stick for five to seven minutes over each point or until the area begins to feel hot.
- ❀ Any ash that forms on the end of the stick can be gently brushed off, using the edge of the ashtray.
- ❀ Never touch the lit end of the moxa stick, even if it looks as if it has gone out.
- ❀ When you have finished, extinguish the stick by placing it lit-end down in your jar, and put the lid on.

When to avoid moxibustion
Avoid moxibustion if there are any signs of Heat or Yin Deficiency, including:

- ❀ night sweating
- ❀ feelings of heat
- ❀ acid indigestion
- ❀ migraines
- ❀ very red tongue on which it looks as if part of the coating is scraped off or peeling.

Reflexology

In reflexology, the two feet together represent the whole body. When treating a client, I imagine a body shape mapped out on the feet, as each organ, gland and nerve has a specific reflex area. The two big toes are the head, the heels are the bottom, with all the parts in between relating to the rest of the body. The outside ankle bones represent the hips and the inside ankle bones correspond to the internal pelvis. Below the inside anklebones, towards the sole, the tissue becomes quite puffy and raised, this is the reflex area for the baby.

As the baby gets bigger in the womb, so does the puffy area on the feet – this bulge can often be more evident on one foot. My advice is to always wear comfortable footwear that gives you support, avoiding tight shoes or socks that leave marks across these reflex areas, as they can become overstimulated.

I will ask you to work in different ways with your fingers. Here are the two main techniques:

✿ Thumb walking or 'caterpillar walking'– so called because the movement of your thumb resembles that of a caterpillar. First, locate the point on the foot to be treated, place your thumb upon it and apply a medium pressure. Move your thumb like a caterpillar as you straighten and bend, applying pressure as you 'walk'.

✿ 'Tornado' – this move is as it sounds. Point your thumb directly downwards, as if drilling a hole, and rotate clockwise and anti-clockwise, exerting a medium pressure.

references

Every effort has been made to contact copyright holders of material reproduced in this book. If any have been inadvertently overlooked, the publishers will be pleased to make restitution at the earliest opportunity.

1. Stadlen, Naomi, *What Mothers Do*, Piatkus, an imprint of Little Brown Book Group 2004.
2. Kaptchuk, Ted, *The Web That Has No Weaver*, Contemporary Books Inc., 2000.
3. In 2008, the *British Medical Journal* online published results they had collated from seven trials carried out in Western countries with a total of 1,366 women. The collated results showed that acupuncture during IVF increased by 65 per cent the change of becoming pregnant, an 87 per cent increase in continuing pregnancy and a 91 per cent increase in live births.
4. Emma Roberts, who contributed the meridian-tapping sections for this book, has thoroughly studied all Gary Craig's educational materials and has personally trained and presented with him. While she feels enormous gratitude and respect for Gary, her views and the author's do not necessarily reflect his or those of EFT. However, we highly recommend the thorough study of the complete and standardized trainings offered at www.emofree.com.
5. The journal *Regulatory, Interface and Comparative Psychology* published a study entitled, 'Effects of acute and chronic sleep on immune modulation of rats' in 2007. Rats were deprived of sleep for twenty-four hours and showed a 20 per cent decrease in white blood cell count, compared with the control group, which is a significant change in the immune system.
6. Mary Jane West-Eberhard quoted in *Mother Nature*.
7. Smoking during pregnancy adversely affects the reproductive systems of male foetuses, according to Scottish scientists, *Journal of Clinical Endocrinology and Metabolism*, 13 November 2007.
8. Harvard School of Public Health in Boston, USA, says that consuming just 4g of trans fats every day can lead to infertility in women.
9. Researchers at the Division of Research, Kaiser Permanente, Northern California, found an increased incidence of miscarriage in women who drank caffeine in the form of coffee, tea, fizzy drinks, hot chocolate or caffeinated soda, compared to women who drank no caffeine. Dr De-Kun Li et al., 'Maternal caffeine consumption during pregnancy and the risk of miscarriage', *American Journal of Obstetrics and Gynecology*, 199(5):e 13–14, November 2008.

10. NICE 2010 guidelines on weight.

11. Cited by Peter Deadman, 'How to be healthy: traditional chinese teachings and modern research', *Journal of Chinese Medicine*, no. 78, June 2005.

12. Rochat de la Vallée, Elizabeth, *Pregnancy and Gestation*, Monkey Press, 2007.

13. Ibid.

14. Australian research has shown acupuncture to be effective in reducing both the severity and incidence of nausea and sickness during pregnancy. This research also followed up on the outcomes for the women involved and concluded that 'acupuncture is a safe and effective treatment for women who experience nausea and dry retching in early pregnancy'. Smith, C., Crowther, C., Beilby, J., 'Acupuncture to treat nausea and vomiting in early pregnancy: a randomized trial', *Birth*, 29 (1):1–9, 2002.

15. A single blind clinical trial carried out in Iran randomly assigned 67 pregnant women to receive either 1,000mg ginger in capsules or placebo capsules for four days. Ginger users demonstrated a higher rate of nausea improvement (85 per cent versus 56 per cent) and a decrease in vomiting (50 per cent versus 9 per cent), *Journal of Alternative Complementary Medicine*, 15(3):243–6, March 2009.

16. Participation in yoga classes can lead to significant reduction in anxiety in women who suffer from anxiety disorders. In the study, women who participated in twice-weekly ninety-minute yoga sessions for two months showed a significant decrease in state and trait anxiety compared to the control group, *Complementary Therapy Clinical Practice*, 15(2):102–4, May 2009.

17. A large American study concluded that acupuncture for back pain results in persistent clinically meaningful improvement, which is better than that achieved with standard care. (A randomized trial comparing acupuncture, simulated acupuncture, and usual care for chronic lower-back pain, *Archives of Internal Medicine*, 11;169(9):858–66, May 2009; in an American trial, one week of continuous auricular acupuncture was shown to decrease the pain and disability experienced by women with pregnancy-related lower-back and posterior-pelvic pain, *American Journal of Obstetrics and Gynecology*, 25 June 2009; research from Sweden concluded that acupuncture was the treatment of choice for symphysis pubis and sacroiliac pain, *British Medical Journal*, 330 (7494):761; Elden, H., et al., 'Effects of acupuncture and stabilizing exercises as adjunct to standard treatment in pregnant women with pelvic-girdle pain: randomized single blind controlled trial', *British Medical Journal*, vol. 330, pp. 761–4, April 2005.

18. Chinese researchers have found acupuncture to be an effective treatment for acute migraine, *Headache*, 49(6):805–16, June 2009.

19. Acupuncture was shown to reduce itching when compared with placebo and non-acupuncture groups, Eleventh Annual Symposium on Complementary Health Care, 2004.

20. Taiwanese researchers have found short-term acupuncture to be as effective as short-term, low-dose prednisolone for mild to moderate carpal-tunnel syndrome, *Clinical Journal of Pain*, 25(4):327–33, May 2009.

21. 'Acupuncture for carpal tunnel syndrome, a systematic review of randomised controlled trials', *Journal of Pain*, 24 November 2010.

22. Lecture notes from RCN Midwifery and Fertility Nursing Forum Conference, p. 11, 5 February 2011.

23. Lewis, J. and Adler, J., 'Forgive and let live', *Newsweek*, 27 September 2004, comparison between individuals in happy relationships and those in unhappy relationships; a 2007 study of ninety-nine participants drew a parallel between forgiveness and lower blood pressure, Robert A. Emmons, *Thanks, how the New Science of gratitude can make you happier*, Houghton Mifflin Harcourt, 2007; a study in 2006 of twenty-five hypertensive patients found forgiveness training reduced their blood pressure, 'Hypertension reduction through forgiveness training', *Journal of Pastoral Care and Counselling* 60 (1–2), 2006 27–34, p. 250 of David Hamilton's book.

24. Researchers in the USA measured foetal responses to a guided meditation designed to induce maternal relaxation during the thirty-second week of pregnancy. The eighteen-minute guided imagery intervention generated significant changes in maternal heart rate, skin conductance, respiration period and respiratory sinus arrhythmia. Significant alterations in foetal behaviour were also observed, including decreased foetal heart rate and suppression of foetal movement, *Biological Psychology*, 31 August 2007.

25. Italian research has demonstrated that moxibustion can have significant effect in helping to turn breech babies. Ideally, treatment is at thirty-four to thirty-five weeks, but can still be used later in pregnancy, *Journal of the American Medical Association*, 280:1580–84; a systematic review from Holland concluded that acupuncture-type interventions are effective in correcting breech presentation, compared with expectant management, *Complementary Therapy Medicine*, 16(2):92–100, April 2008.

26. Acupuncture treatment given weekly from three to four weeks prior to due date to prepare the pelvis and cervix for labour has been shown by a New Zealand study with midwives to reduce the need for medical intervention, including medical induction and Caesarean section, *Medical Acupuncture*, Vol. 17, No. 3, 2006.

27. 'Postnatal Care – Still a Cinderella Story?' findings of an NCT survey of first-time mothers and the case for change, October 2010.

28. Erlewein, Rebecca, 'Congee – Food for life', *Journal of Chinese Medicine*, No. 92, February 2010.

29. Gerhardt, Sue, *Why Love Matters*, Routledge, 2004.

resources

Useful Contacts
Emma Cannon
www.emmacannon.co.uk
Telephone: 07531 916 121
Chelsea Outpatient Centre
280 Kings Road, London SW1W 8RH

137 Harley Street, London W1G 6BF

Within the practice, we offer an integrated approach to fertility and pregnancy, gynaecology and family health. We offer acupuncture, antenatal classes, fertility tests, fertility and IVF support and reflexology; we work closely with many like-minded practitioners, both in the fields of Western and complementary therapies.
Acupuncturists: Kate Freemantle, Laura Hersch, Camilla Festing
Reflexology: Joanna Spriggs and Laura Hersch
Fertility nurse: Lynne Ager RGNONC
Midwife: Anna Cannon RMPGdipIAIM LC

I also have a satellite clinic at The Birth Company
www.thebirthcompany.co.uk

British Acupuncture Council
This is the UK's main regulatory body for the practice of traditional acupuncture by over 2,400 acupuncturists.
www.acupuncture.org.uk
Telephone: 020 8735 0400
63 Jeddo Road, London W12 9HQ

FSID (The Foundation for the Study of Infant Deaths)
A charity working to prevent sudden infant deaths.
www.fsid.org.uk
Telephone: 020 7802 3200
Helpline: 080 8802 6868
11 Belgrave Road
London SW1V 1RB

General Osteopathic Council
www.osteopathy.org.uk
Telephone: 020 7357 6655
176 Tower Bridge Road
London SE1 3LU

NICE (National Institute for Clinical Excellence)
An independent organization responsible for providing national guidance on
promoting good health and preventing ill health.
www.nice.org.uk
Telephone: 0845 003 7780
MidCity Place
71 High Holborn
London WC1V 6NA

The Register of Chinese Herbal Medicine
A register set up to regulate the practice of Chinese Herbal Medicine in the UK.
www.rchm.co.uk
Telephone: 01603 623994
Office 5, 1 Exeter Street
Norwich NR2 4QB

Sands (Stillbirth & Neonatal Death Charity)
www.uk-sands.org
National Helpline: 020 7436 5881
28 Portland Place
London W1B 1LY

More Information about Pre- and Postnatal Care

AcuMedic

A Chinese medicine supplier where you can buy books, charts ear-press seeds and moxibustion supplies.

www.acumedic.com

Telephone: 020 7388 6704

101–105 Camden High Street

London NW1 7JN

BFN (The Breastfeeding Network)

PO Box 11126

Paisley PA2 8YB

Support line: 0300 100 0210

www.breastfeedingnetwork.org.uk

La Leche League

www.laleche.org.uk

Breastfeeding helpline: 0845 456 1855

PO Box 29

West Bridgford

Nottingham

NG2 7NP

LCGB (Lactation Consultants of Great Britain)

Find your nearest lactation consultant through this organization.

www.lcgb.org

National Childbirth Trust

www.nct.org.uk

Telephone: 0300 330 0770

Alexandra House

Oldham Terrace

London W3 6NH

Neals Yard Remedies

For information on essential oils and some herbs.
www.nealsyardremedies.com
Telephone: 0845 262 3145
NYR Direct
Peacemarsh, Gillingham
Dorset SP8 4EU

Oxford Medical Supplies

Sells moxibustion supplies.
www.oxfordmedical.co.uk
Telephone: 0800 975 8000
Units 11 & 12, Horcott Industrial Estate
Fairford, Gloucestershire GL7 4BX

Organic Box Schemes

www.riverford.co.uk
www.abelandcole.co.uk

Private Pregnancy

A resource for mums-to-be in the UK who wish to look at private health-care for fertility, IVF, maternity care, pregnancy scans and childbirth related services.
www.PrivatePregnancy.co.uk

Useful Websites

Acupressure for natural pain relief in labour DVD by Debra Betts and Tom Kennedy
www.jcm.co.uk
www.acupuncture.rhizome.net.nz/acupressure-intro.aspx

www.duofertility.com for fertility monitoring

MamaTENS (for pain relief during labour)
www.mama-tens.info
(also email: help@mama-tens.info; telephone: 01372 723 434)
www.mooncup.co.uk (for more information on the alternative to tampons)

Simon and Sally Givertz
www.learn-shiatsu.org.uk (for a full visual guide to the Eight Strands of the
Brocade visit www.learn-shiatsu.org.uk/EightTreasuresCourseMaterial.pdf)

www.smokefree.nhs.uk (for help with quitting smoking)
www.nhs.uk/livewell/drugs (for information and help with quitting drugs)

Recommended Relaxation Resources

Yogabirth 1, Sitaram, available from www.sitaram.org
Yoga nidra (deep relaxation) from DVD 1 in *Mother Nurture: Gentle Yoga for
the Transition to Motherhood*, Sitaram, available from www.sitaram.org
Mother's Breath, a triple audio CD set from Sitaram Yoga, www.sitaram.org.

Practitioners

Anna Cannon LC

Independent midwife and lactation consultant. For all your midwifery needs in
the comfort of your own home, including antenatal appointments, labour care,
home births, postnatal care and baby massage for individuals or small groups.
Email: annacannon@btinternet.com
Telephone: 07891 570113
www.annacannon.co.uk

Kate Cook BA Hons, Dip ION, MBANT

Nutritional therapist, director of The Nutrition Coach and author of several
books on nutrition.
www.thenutritioncoach.co.uk
Email: kate@thenutritioncoach.co.uk
Telephone: 0845 050 2442

The Nutrition Coach at The Birth Company
137 Harley Street
London W1G 6BG

Mr William Dennes

Mr William Dennes is a Consultant Obstetrician and Sub-specialist in Maternal and Foetal Medicine. He is a Consultant at King's College Hospital, London. He works both in the NHS and privately, looking after mothers at both King's College Hospital (the Guthrie Wing) and the Portland Hospital. Mr Dennes is experienced in the management of women in pregnancy, and has a special interest in multiple pregnancies and high-risk obstetric cases.
The Women's Health Partnership
30 Devonshire Street
London W1G 6PU
Telephone: 020 7486 2440

Uma Dinsmore-Tuli

Yoga teacher and author based in London who specializes in fertility, pregnancy and postnatal yoga.
www.sitaram.org
Telephone: 07595 219759

Dr Donald Gibb

Consultant obstetrician, The Birth Company: a leading women's pregnancy care, childbirth and gynaecology clinic based in Harley Street, London.
www.thebirthcompany.co.uk
Telephone: 020 7725 0528
137 Harley Street
London W1G 6BF

Maxine Hamilton-Stubber

Osteopath, chiropractor and physiotherapist
www.maxosteopaths.com
Telephone: 020 7730 7928 (Weds and Fri); 020 7631 3276 (Thurs)

Daverick Leggett

Shiatsu practitioner, qigong teacher and author of several Chinese dietary books. All Daverick's work is available at www.meridianpress.net.
PO Box 3
Totnes
Devon TQ9 5WJ

Emma Roberts

Pioneer of EFT and Meridian Tapping in the UK; she runs the EFT Centre with Sue Beer.
www.theeftcentre.com

Jacquelyn Schirmer

Osteopath/Pilates and pre/postnatal teacher.
Telephone: 07957553222
Email: jacschirmer@hotmail.com
Guild of Pregnancy and Postnatal Exercise Teachers
www.postnatalexercise.co.uk

Sossi Yerissian

Nutrition consultancy and Manual Lymphatic Drainage (MLD) Therapy.
53 New Cavendish Street, London W1G 9TQ
Telephone: 07815 633 628
www.sossi.co.uk
(MLD UK – PO Box 14491, Glenroths, Fife, Scotland KY6 3YE
telephone: 08448 001 988; www.mlduk.org.uk)

Miss Jeannie Yoon

Consultant obstetrician and gynaecologist.
132 Harley Street
London W1G YJX

The Lister Hospital, Chelsea Bridge Road
London SW1W 8RH
Telephone: 020 7730 2383

Kathleen Beegun
www.yogabirth.org

The Qigong Institute
Promotes qigong and energy medicine through research and education.
www.qigonginstitute.org

further reading

Harriet Beinfield and Efrem Korngold, *Between Heaven and Earth: A Guide to Chinese Medicine*, Ballantine Books, 1992.

Debra Betts, *The Essential Guide to Acupuncture in Pregnancy & Childbirth*, Journal of Chinese Medicine, 2006.

Sarah Blaffer Hardy, *Mother Nature*, Chatto & Windus, 1999.

Linda Chih-Ling Koo, *Nourishment of Life: Health in Chinese Society*, Commercial Press, 1982.

Lorraine Clissold, *Why the Chinese Don't Count Calories*, Constable, 2008.

Sue Cox, *Breastfeeding with Confidence: a Practical Guide*, Meadowbrook Press, 2006.

Anita Diamant, *The Red Tent*, Pan, 2002.

Rebecca Erlewein, 'Congee – longevity food for life', *Journal of Chinese Medicine*, number 92, February 2010.

Uma Dinsmore-Tuli, *Mother's Breath*, Hodder, 2006.

Uma Dinsmore-Tuli, *Teach Yourself Yoga for Pregnancy and Birth*, Hodder, 2007.

Bob Flaws, *Arisal of the Clear*, Blue Poppy Press, 1991.

Bob Flaws and Honora Wolfe, *Prince Wen Hui's Cook: Chinese Dietary Therapy*, Paradigm Publications, 1983.

Ina May Gaskin, *Ina May's Guide to Childbirth*, Vermilion, 2008.

Sue Gerhardt, *Why Love Matters: How Affection Shapes a Baby's Brain*, Routledge, 2004.

David R. Hamilton RhD, *Why Kindness is Good for You*, Hay House, 2010.

Angela Hicks, *The Five Laws for Healthy Living*, Thorsons, 1998.

Ted Kaptchuk, *The Web That Has No Weaver*, Contemporary Books Inc., 2000.

La Leche League International, *The Womanly Art of Breastfeeding*, Pinter & Martin Ltd, 2010.

Daverick Leggett, *Helping Ourselves: Guide to Traditional Chinese Food Energetics*, Meridian Press, 1994.

Daverick Leggett, *Recipes for Self-Healing*, Meridian Press, 1999.

Nancy Mohrbacher and Kathleen A. Kendell-Tackett, *Breastfeeding Made Simple*, New Harbinger Publications, 2010.

Gowri Motha, *The Gentle Birth Method*, Thorsons, 2004.

Michel Odent, *The Caesarean*, Free Association Books, 1988.

Professor Lesley Regan, *Miscarriage – What Every Woman Needs to Know*, Orion, 1997.

Elisabeth Rochat de la Vallée, *Pregnancy and Gestation*, Monkey Press, 2007.

Joe Simpson, *Touching the Void*, Vintage, 1998.

Naomi Stadlen, *What Mothers Do: Especially When It Looks Like Nothing*, Piatkus Books, 2004.

The Journal of Chinese Medicine (www.jcm.co.uk).

index

acknowledgements

Thank you to everyone who has helped me. It takes a lot of energy to create a book, and by helping me you have helped me to help others.

To Kate Adams for being a dream writing partner. To Clare Hulton, my agent, for being fantastic at things I am not. To Liz Gough for commissioning me in the first place and giving me the chance to be an author. To Cindy Chan and everyone at Pan Macmillan, from marketing to sales and everyone in between; it is thrilling being involved in such a creative process. To Tamara Ellis for the cover illustration, Juliet Percival for the illustrations inside, Jonathan Baker for the perfect layout design and to Anne Newman and Gill Paul for their copy-editing skills. Thank you also Brigid Moss and Emma Draude for your communications skills and Claire Norrish for spreading the word.

To Tim Evans for believing in my approach and helping me get my practice started all those years ago. To Jeannie Yoon for your support in my approach and your immense skill as a practitioner. To John Tindall for your support of my practice and of my health. To Peta Martin for your love and support.

To my team: Michelle Mazewski, Kate Freemantle, Laura Hersch and Camilla Festing; I could not do it without you. To Donald Gibb for your support, the kind foreword to this book and for providing me with such a wonderful and calm place to work from. Thank you also to William Dennes for medically checking the book. To Anna Cannon, for your incredible skill as a midwife and for bringing my two children safely into the world and now for helping me to bring this book to life – you are a true facilitator of life. To Emma Roberts, your work makes my work with people so much easier; you are an amazing person. To Uma Dinsmore-Tuli for your ability to flow gently in and out of my life, always being there with the right message at the right time (unknowingly), making sure I am not straying off my path, and for the beautiful yoga in this book. To Maxine Hamilton-Stubber, Kate Cook, Joanna Spriggs, Sossi Yerissian, Kathleen Beegan and Jacqui Schirmer for your unique skills and your generosity of spirit. Thank you all for your part in this book – the pages are full of your wisdom. And to my oldest friend

Danielle Margulies for helping me create the nourishing recipes in this book – it has been such a bonus doing this with you.

Thank you to Debra Betts, Sarah Budd, Daverick Leggett and Jani White for your work in Chinese medicine that has helped raise the standards in this area and influenced my practice.

To Sophie Dahl for your mouth-watering recipe.

To my family Roger, Lily and Violet for knowing I needed to follow my heart and giving me the space to do it.

Finally a thanks to my wonderful patients; I am so blessed to do the work that I do and to be involved in the fine-tuning of your bodies and trusted with your hopes and dreams. I am learning from you every day and your stories never cease to move me.